Happy Food Cookbook

Kimber Reese, Chef

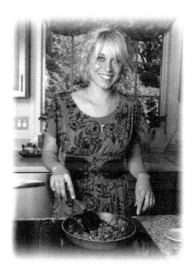

All Happy Food recipes are free of gluten, processed sugar, butter, corn, canola oil and soy and many are vegetarian or vegan!

"Let thy food be thy medicine, and thy medicine be thy food."
-Hippocrates

> *This cookbook and the recipes contained within are not intended as a substitute for the advice or medical care of a physician.*
>
> *Any person with chronic illness or disease should consult with a physician before beginning any nutrition or lifestyle program.*
>
> *If the reader has any questions or concerns about the recipes or ingredients presented in this book, or its application to any particular medical profile, or if the reader has any unusual medical conditions or food allergies, he or she should consult the advice of their physician.*

All photography by Yolanda Ciolli, used with permission.

ISBN 978-1-942168-16-4

Published by Compass Flower Press
an imprint of AKA-Publishing
Columbia, MO
CompassFlowerPress.com

To Gramma,
an inspiring force in my life.

Introduction

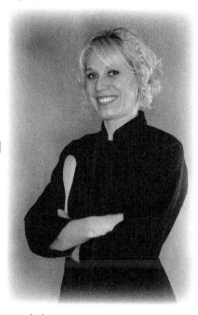

I was driving home from a yoga teacher training in a car full of teachers when I was asked, "What do you eat?"

I tried to explain it—the simplicity, the ease, the health reasons, the cooking techniques, and I could tell it was new to them all.

They asked if I could write some recipes for them. Since I never wrote any recipes down, I decided to write a cookbook.

I wanted to share my knowledge of cooking, baking and nutrition that fostered the way I eat. I wanted to create a cookbook that was true to the way I eat, which I believe can help people with health issues, allergies and the effort to lose weight.

My goal with the Happy Food Cookbook is to educate people in anyway I can to help them eat healthier delicious food without the guilt or negative affects of processed foods.

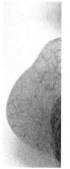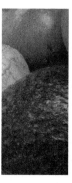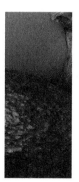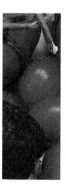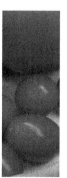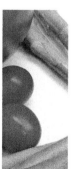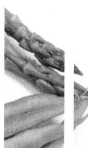

CONTENTS

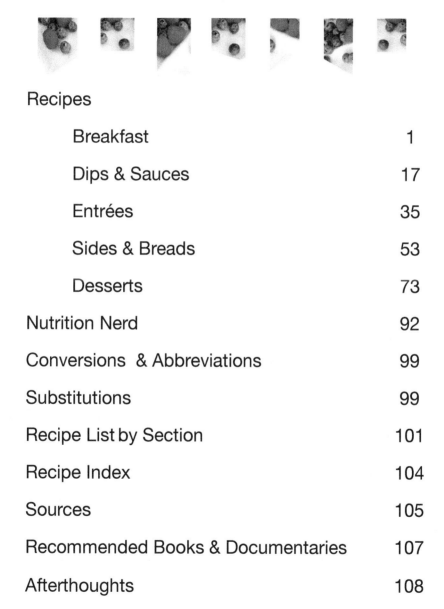

BREAKFAST

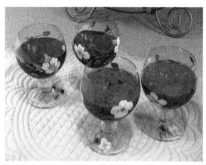 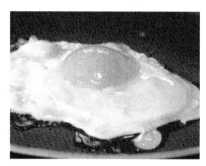

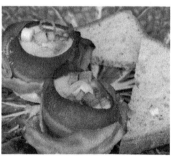 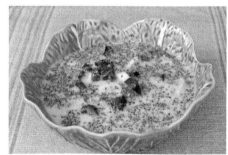

Berry Breakfast Smoothie

Preparation Time: 5 minutes
Cook Time: 0 minutes
Yield: 1 smoothie

I like to add a tablespoon of: spirulina, bee pollen, hemp protein powder and maca powder. It's instant energy. Great as an on-the-go breakfast.

1 banana
1/2 cup orange juice
1/2 cup blueberries
1/2 cup raspberries
1/4 cup plain Greek yogurt

1. Place everything into a blender. Mix until smooth. Enjoy!

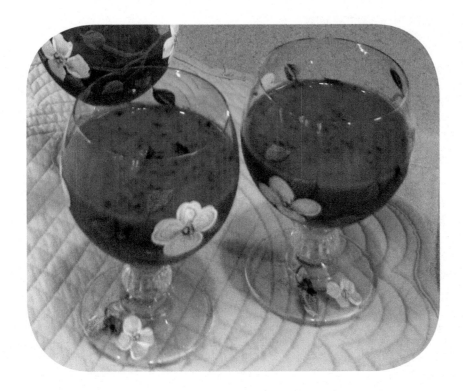

Peanut Butter Yum

Preparation Time: 8 minutes
Cook Time: 0 minutes
Yield: 1 smoothie

To make this vegetarian or vegan, substitute almond yogurt, ice or more dark chocolate almond milk for the Greek yogurt.

1/2 cup dark chocolate almond milk
2 dates
1 banana
1/4 cup plain Greek yogurt
2 tablespoons creamy peanut butter
1/2 tablespoon cacao powder
1/2 tablespoon maca powder
1/2 cup blueberries

1. Add all ingredients to a blender. Mix well, and welcome to a little piece of heaven.

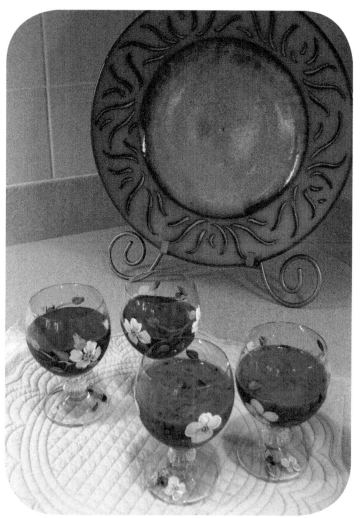

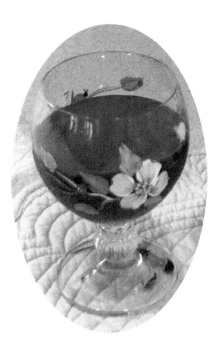

Avocado Toast

Preparation Time: 5 minutes
Cook Time: 3 minutes
Yield: 1 serving

Quick, easy and full of sustainable energy.

1 slice **Kimber's Healthy Gluten-free Bread (p. 59)**
1/2 avocado, Leave as the full half and scoop out of skin
1 slice tomato
1 teaspoon extra virgin olive oil
1 egg
1 teaspoon hot sauce
1 pinch salt and pepper

1. Toast the slice of bread.
2. Place tomato slice on toasted bread. Halve the avocado and place it with the seed removed side up, on top of the tomato slice.
3. Heat the pan with extra virgin olive oil to medium heat. Crack the egg into the pan and let cook for a few minutes. Coagulate and flip egg, and cook for 30 seconds. Remove from heat, place fried egg in the middle of avocado where the pit use to be. Drizzle hot sauce on top and add salt and pepper to taste.

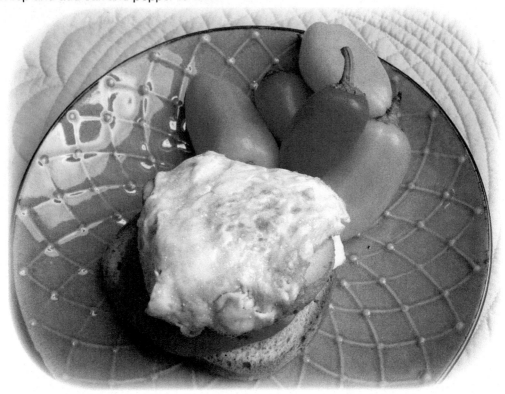

Berry Tart

Preparation Time: 15 minutes
Cook Time: 0 minutes
Yield: 10-12 servings

I eat this raw but it is delicious baked at 325 for 18 minutes as well. Eat warm.

2 cups raw walnuts
1 cup soft, pitted, about 9 dates
1 tablespoon almond flour
2 tablespoons honey

1 pint quartered strawberries
1 pint blueberries
2 tablespoons almond flour
3/4 cup peach jam
2 tablespoons chia seeds
2 tablespoons Coconut Oil

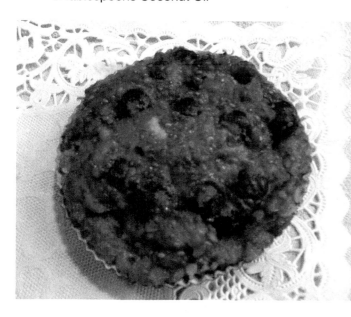

1. Grease tart pan. Place walnuts, almond flour, honey and dates in food processor and blend until smooth.
2. Add 1-3 tsp of water until the dough has a texture that stays together.
3. Press crust into the bottom and sides of the pan.
4. In a bowl mix in the peach jam, chia seeds, coconut oil and almond flour. Mix in the berries until it is all coated. Pour and spread over tart crust.
5. Serve immediately and store in an air-tight container in the refrigerator.

Baked Veggie Mini-Frittata

Preparation Time: 10 minutes
Cook Time: 14-16 minutes
Yield: 10-12 quiches

3 eggs
1/2 can drained, rinsed black beans
1/2 cup cauliflower
4 mushrooms
1/2 cup zucchini
3 tablespoons cilantro
2 tablespoons unsweetened almond milk
1/2 teaspoon black pepper
1/2 cup Kale
3 dashes hot sauce
1/4 cup asiago cheese
1/2 carrot
1 teaspoon salt

1. Preheat oven to 400 and spray muffin liners.
2. Blend all ingredients in a food processor or blender.
3. Fill muffin tins 2/3 of the way full. Bake for 14-16 minutes. Top with **Creamy Avocado Sauce (p. 23)** or **Urban Pico De Gallo Salsa (p. 21)**. Enjoy!

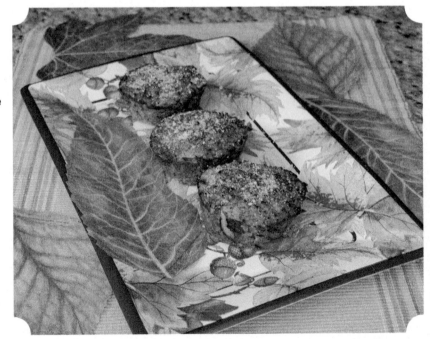

Oatmeal Peanut Butter Breakfast Bars

Preparation Time: 10 minutes
Cook Time: 18-20 minutes
Yield: 20 bars

To make this raw, make exactly the same, but leave it in the fridge overnight. To make vegan switch the honey to agave.

1/2 cup **Quick and Easy Fresh Applesauce (p. 89)**
3 soft dates
3/4 cup peanut butter
1/2 cup honey
1 tablespoon oat bran
2 cups rolled oats
1/4 cup slivered almonds
1/4 cup raisins
1/4 cup chopped dried apples

1. Grease a 9x11 pan and preheat oven to 325.
2. Mash dates and mix well with **Quick and Easy Fresh Applesauce (p. 89)**. Add peanut butter and honey and mix.
3. Add oat bran and oats. Mix well. Fold in almonds, raisins, and dried apples.
4. Press into pregreased pan.
5. Bake for 18-20 minutes, until a toothpick comes out clean.

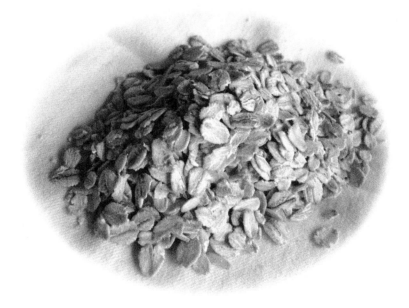

Banana Date Chia Cereal

Preparation Time: 8 minutes
Cook Time: 0 minutes
Yield: 1 serving

If you don't eat bananas any berry is a great substitute.

1/4 cup chia seeds
1 cup unsweetened vanilla almond milk
1/2 cup chopped dates
1/2 sliced banana

1. In a cereal bowl, add chia seeds and milk. Stir so the chia seeds don't clump.
2. Add prepared dates and banana and let sit for 5 minutes.
3. Eat up!

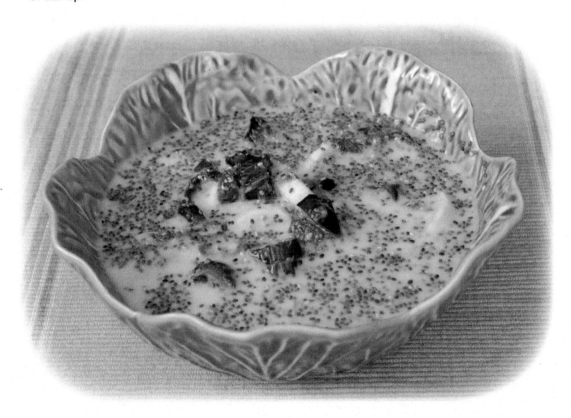

French Toast Sticks

Preparation Time: 1 minutes
Cook Time: 16-18 minutes
Yield: 15 sticks

15 sticks 1"x 3" **Kimber's Healthy Gluten-free Bread (p. 59)**
2 tablespoons flax meal
6 tablespoons water
1/2 cup unsweetened almond milk
1 tablespoon agave
1/2 teaspoon ground cinnamon
1 teaspoon vanilla extract
2 1/2 cups crushed banana chips or granola

1. Grease two 13x9 pans.
2. Cut bread into sticks. Place in a single layer in greased pan.
3. Use a Ziploc bag to place the banana chips in and mash with a rolling pin or use a food processor. You also can use your favorite granola, no mashing necessary.
4. With a fork mix together flax meal and water. Add milk, agave, cinnamon and vanilla, and mix well. Pour over the bread sticks and allow to sit for 2 minutes, then flip to make sure both sides are coated, let sit another 2 minutes.
5. Coat the soaked bread sticks by rolling them in the crumble in a bowl. Place in the other

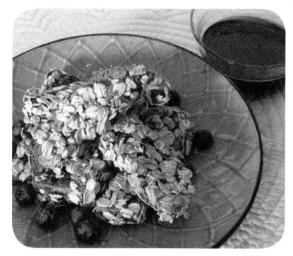

prepared dish, leaving space for better airflow while cooking.
6. Place sticks in the pan with the top covered for 45 minutes to overnight in the freezer.
7. When ready to bake, preheat oven to 425 and bake for 16-18 minutes. Eat with syrup, **Easy Strawberry Jam (p. 28)**, **Easy Peach Jam (p. 28)**, or your favorite toppings.

Asiago Kale Scramble

Preparation Time: 5 minutes
Cook Time: 10 minutes
Yield: 1 serving

2 cups chopped Kale
2 tablespoons extra virgin olive oil
1/4 cup jalapeño slices (from jar)
1/2 diced avocado
1/4 cup salsa
2 eggs
2 tablespoons grated asiago cheese

1. Put extra virgin olive oil, kale and jalapeños in cold sauté pan and turn on med-high heat, sauté.
2. Add eggs directly to pan and stir into the kale mixture until scrambled.
3. Take off heat and place in a serving bowl.
4. Top with avocado, salsa and cheese.

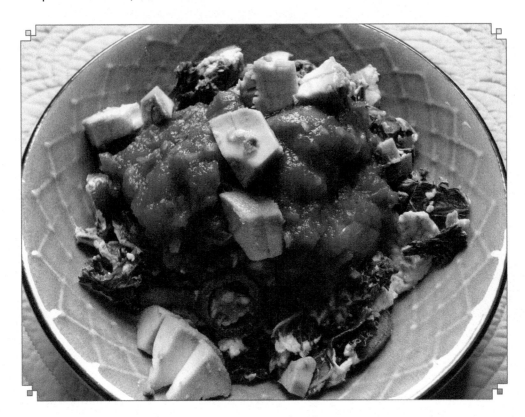

Kale Hummus Breakfast/Knish

Preparation Time: 5 minutes
Cook Time: 10 minutes
Yield: 1 serving

I eat this raw most mornings. I feel better eating it raw, but I still love this cooked.

2 cups chopped, cleaned Kale
2 tablespoons extra virgin olive oil
2 tablespoons jalapeño slices (from jar)
1/4 cup **Lemon Garlic Hummus (p. 27)**
1/3 avocado, diced
1/4 cup salsa
1/3 cup raw almonds

1. Place extra virgin olive oil, kale and jalapeños in sautée pan while cold and turn to med-high heat. Sauté until kale is translucent, about 5-8 minutes.
2. Add hummus to coat and cook until heated through, about 4 minutes.
3. Put into a bowl. Add avocado, almonds and salsa. Eat warm.

Knish:
After sautéing the kale and jalapeños, add the hummus. You want to start spreading the hummus so that all the kale is incorporated. Once the hummus begins to heat through it is easier for the kale to incorporate. Then push the hummus and kale patty flat like a pancake and let each side get lightly browned, so the patty holds better. You can make small ones, but I like one big Knish on my plate. Top with salsa, avocado and cheese and enjoy!

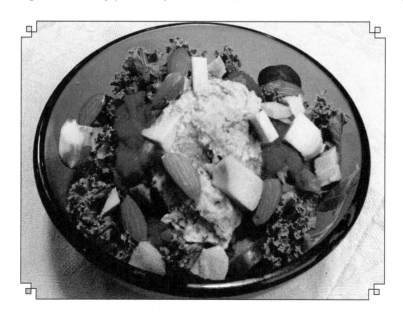

Chocolate Protein Oatmeal

Preparation Time: 3 minutes
Cook Time: 7 minutes
Yield: 1 serving

Favorite winter breakfast to warm my soul. You can also soak the oats and chocolate almond milk overnight in a mason jar to keep them raw. Add the rest of the ingredients in the morning and eat cold.

1/4 cup rolled oats
1/2 cup dark chocolate almond milk
1 teaspoon flax meal
1 scoop your favorite brand chocolate protein
1/4 cup raisins

1. In pot add almond milk and bring to a boil. Add oats and flax meal, reduce to a simmer for 5 minutes uncovered. Remove from heat. Let stand 2 minutes.
2. Mix protein powder into the oats well. Add raisins and mix. Eat warm.

If using a microwave heat oats, flax meal and almond milk for 90 seconds. No need to let stand before mixing protein powder in. Add raisins once all other ingredients are combined.

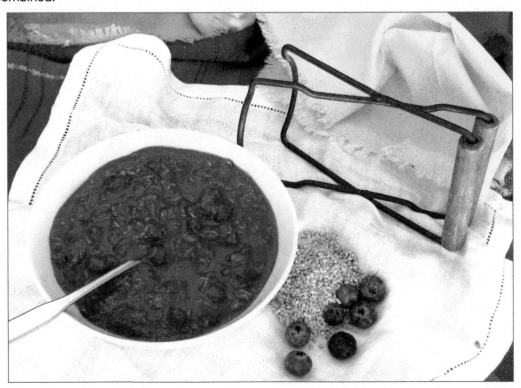

Morning Glory Muffins

Preparation Time: 25 minutes
Cook Time: 28-32 minutes or until the bottom and side of the muffins are golden brown.
Yield: 24 muffins

3/4 cup honey
3 tablespoons flax meal
6 tablespoons water
1 cup **Quick and Easy Fresh Applesauce (p. 89)**
2 teaspoons vanilla extract
2 1/4 cups brown rice flour
1 teaspoon guar gum
1 tablespoon ground cinnamon
2 teaspoons baking soda
1 tablespoon baking powder
1/2 teaspoon salt
2 cups grated carrots
1 grated apple
8 ounces drained, crushed pineapple
3/4 cup raisins
1/2 cup shredded coconut
1/2 cup chopped pecans

1. Preheat oven to 350. Grease muffin liners. In a small bowl and a fork mix flax meal and water together.
2. In a large bowl or kitchen aid, mix honey, **Quick and Easy Fresh Applesauce (p. 89)**, flax meal mixture and vanilla until well combined.
3. In a separate bowl mix flour, guar gum, cinnamon, salt, baking soda and baking powder with a dry fork. Slowly add dry ingredients to the wet ingredients, about 1/3 at a time. Only mix until incorporated, still a little lumpy.
4. Add carrots, apples, pineapple, raisins, coconut and pecans and fold into batter.
5. Spoon into muffin tins about 3/4 of the way full. Bake for 25-30 minutes or until a toothpick comes out clean.

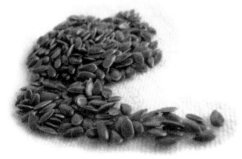

Nutty Protein Pancakes

Preparation Time: 5 minutes
Cook Time: 12 minutes
Yield: 1 serving

1 cup peanut butter
1/4 cup **Quick and Easy Fresh Applesauce (p. 89)**
2 tablespoons flaxseed
1/2 cup raisins
1 egg
1/2 teaspoon vanilla extract
1/4 teaspoon ground cinnamon

1. Heat a griddle to low-med heat.
2. Mix peanut butter, **Quick and Easy Fresh Applesauce (p. 89)**, egg and flax seeds together on a bowl.
3. Add vanilla and cinnamon, mix.
4. Mix in raisins.
5. Pour batter onto griddle and cook on each side for about 4-6 minutes, until golden brown. If really thick you can add 1-2 tbsp of water, just watch the cooking time.

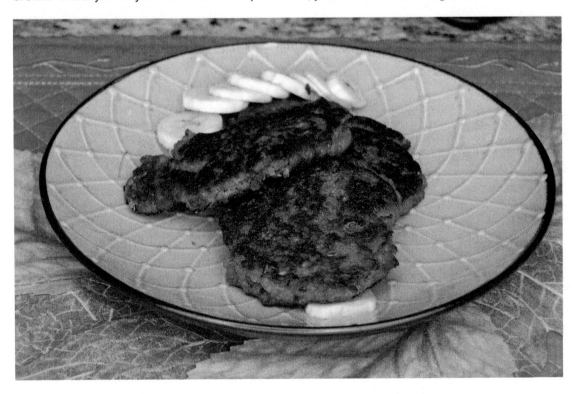

Bacon & Egg Club Cups

Preparation Time: 5 minutes
Cook Time: 12 minutes
Yield: 1 serving (double recipe for a hungry morning)

Every man's dream breakfast. Fast, easy and full of lean protein.

1 slice turkey bacon
1 slice turkey or your favorite deli meat
1 egg
1 tablespoon grated Parmesan cheese
1 dash hot pepper sauce
1 teaspoon sliced scallions

1. Preheat oven to 400 and grease one muffin tin.
2. Line muffin tin with slice of turkey around the bottom and sides. Over that, line the sides of the same tin with turkey bacon. You now have two kinds of meat for lining.
3. Crack egg into middle of meat cup and add a dash of hot sauce on top. Bake for 12 minutes.
4. Remove from muffin tin and place on a plate. Top with cheese and green onions. Serve warm.

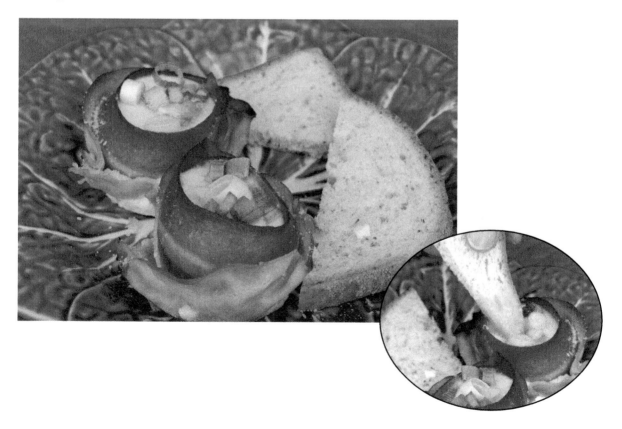

Pumpkin Chocolate Chip Waffles

Preparation Time: 10 minutes
Cook Time: 10-13 minutes
Yield: 3 servings

1 1/2 cup pumpkin puree
1/2 cup **Quick and Easy Fresh Applesauce (p. 89)**
1 teaspoon ground nutmeg
2 teaspoon ground cinnamon
2 teaspoon vanilla extract
2 egg
6 tablespoons flax meal
2 cup almond flour
1 cup **Kimber's Chocolate (p. 59)**

1. Preheat your waffle iron while making the batter. Make sure to spray iron with nonstick spray every time you add new batter to the iron.
2. Mix pumpkin puree and **Quick and Easy Fresh Applesauce (p. 89)** together in a bowl. Add egg and vanilla, mix well.
3. In a smaller separate bowl, mix almond flour, cinnamon, nutmeg and flax meal together. Pour into wet ingredients and mix until incorporated.
4. Fold in chocolate chips.
5. Spray heated waffle iron and add enough batter to fill each waffle space. Cook for 10-13 minutes. Enjoy!

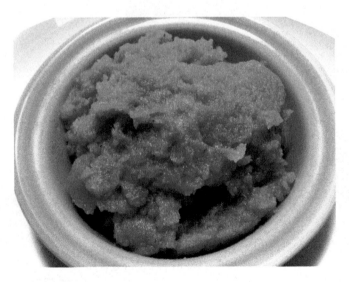
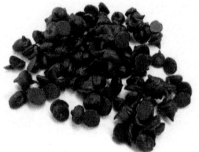

DIPS & SAUCES

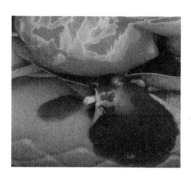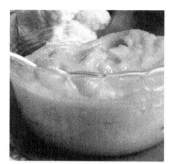

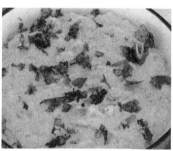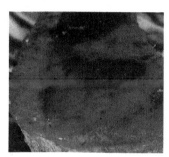

Favorite Berry Sauce

Preparation Time: 5 minutes
Cook Time: 20 minutes
Yield: 12 ounces

If I use strawberries, I half them before I cook them.

16 ounces (1 pint) berries: any of your favorite berries work
1/4 cup maple syrup
1/2 lemon juice
1/2 grated green apples

1. Place all ingredients into a sauce pan. Bring to a boil, then reduce to medium heat for 20 minutes. Stirring occasionally.
2. You can leave chunky or use a blender or food processor to smooth out. Serve warm or cold.

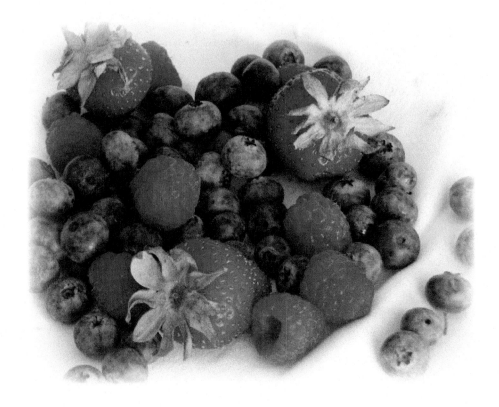

Over 21 BBQ Sauce

Preparation Time: 5 minutes
Cook Time: 0 minutes
Yield: 1 pint

I use all my home made jams and ketchup. Use whichever you like, the peach jam is a nice taste as well. I also use the gluten free beer, Omission Beer (which doesn't contain high fructose corn syrup) or a good lager that is widely available.

3/4 cup **Best Home Made Ketchup (p. 26)**
1/4 cup **Easy strawberry Jam (p. 28)**
1/2 cup Worcestershire sauce
1/4 cup Omission Gluten Free Beer
1 teaspoon minced garlic

1. Mix all ingredients in a bowl. Amazing!

Pictured below on **Simple BBQ Chicken Grill (p. 42)**

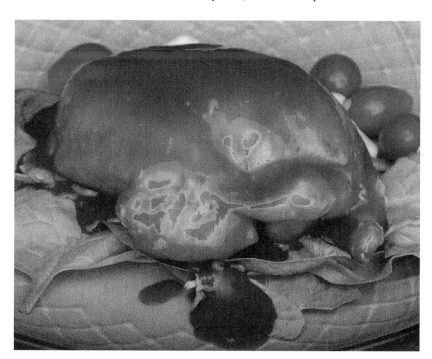

Hot Chili Hummus

Preparation Time: 15 minutes
Cook Time: 0 minutes
Yield: 1 quart

This hummus is full of spices that remind me of my favorite chili recipe. The acidity of the tomatoes is a wonderful flavor as well. It's spicy, but feel free to add more hot sauce or jalapeños to turn up the heat!

1 can garbanzo beans
1 (15-ounce) container sesame tahini
1/2 cup grape seed oil
½ pint or 8 oz packages cherry tomatoes
1 tablespoon ground cumin
3 tablespoons chili powder
1 teaspoon black pepper
1 teaspoon ground paprika
1 tablespoon minced, dried garlic
1 teaspoon Tabasco Hot Sauce
3/4 cup diced jalapeños
1/4 sliced red onion

1. Drain garbanzo beans, keep the juice! Add beans and tahini to food processor and pulse for 30 seconds.
2. Add grape seed oil, onion and tomatoes, turn on for 10 seconds.
3. Add cumin, chili powder, pepper, paprika, garlic, and hot sauce. Turn on for 10 seconds, then keep it on and slowly drizzle in the garbanzo bean juice.
4. Turn off, wipe down the sides and turn on until everything is incorporated. Scrape into a bowl. Mix in jalapeños.
5. Serve warm or cold, store in the refrigerator.

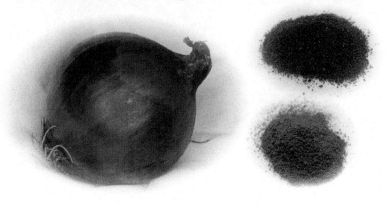

Urban Pico de Gallo Salsa

Preparation Time: 10 minutes
Cook Time: 0 minutes
Yield: 8 servings

This salsa is fresh, chunky and full of flavor that reminds me of chili.

6 medium, diced tomatoes
2 tablespoons minced garlic
1 medium, diced red onion
1/2 juice lime
1/4 cup chopped cilantro
1 cup jalapeño slices, (from jar) roughly chopped
1 tablespoon ground cumin

1. Place tomatoes, onion, jalapeños and garlic in a large bowl.
2. Add lime juice and cumin and stir well.
3. Add chopped cilantro and give a light stir. You can save a couple cilantro leaves as a garnish for the top if you'd like. Great with chips or on eggs.

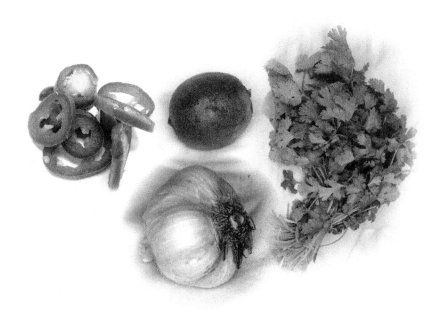

Tart Cranberry Sauce

Preparation Time: 10 minutes
Cook Time: 10 minutes
Yield: 1 pint

If this recipe is too tart for your taste buds, add some maple syrup to sweeten it up.

1 cup water
12 ounces cranberries
1/2 cup molasses
2 teaspoons minced ginger
1 juiced orange

1. In a saucepan add all ingredients and bring to a boil. Simmer for 10 minutes. Serve warm or cold. I love this dish at Thanksgiving.

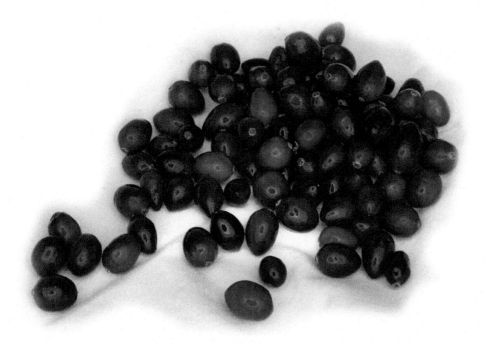

Creamy Avocado Sauce

Preparation Time: 8 minutes
Cook Time: 0 minutes
Yield: 1 pint

2 ripe avocados
1/4 cup coconut milk
1/3 cup vegetable broth
1/2 cup packed parsley or 2 tbsp. dried parsley
1/3 cup extra virgin olive oil
1 juiced, zested lime
1 tablespoon minced garlic
2 teaspoons ground cumin

1. Add all ingredients into food processor and blend until smooth. Add more broth to smooth out if too stiff.

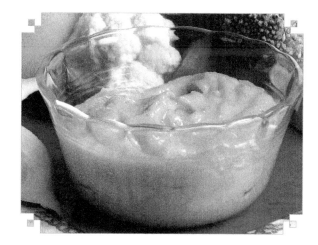

Smooth & Mild Guacamole

Preparation Time: 10 minutes
Cook Time: 0 minutes
Yield: 1-2 pints

3 avocados
1 medium, diced tomato
1/4 diced red onion
1 tablespoon minced garlic
1/4 cup plain Greek yogurt
1/2 teaspoon black pepper
1/2 teaspoon sea salt
1/2 teaspoon cumin
3 dashes Tabasco hot sauce

1. Mash avocados. I use my hands, but the back of a fork or a potato masher works well too.
2. Add the yogurt and mix.
3. Add the rest of the ingredients. Add more of anything to fit your taste buds.

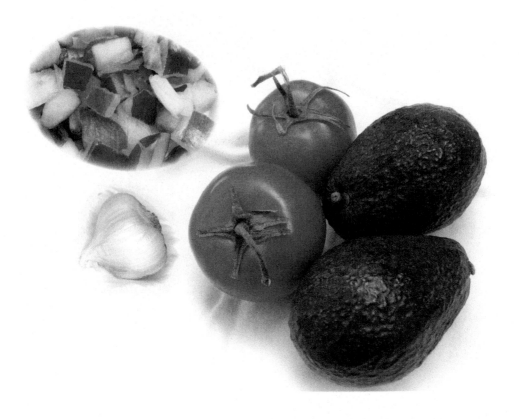

Lemon Honey Dijon Dressing

Preparation Time: 10 minutes
Cook Time: 0 minutes
Yield: 1 pint

Add sea salt if you like salt. It will change the flavor and sometimes I do it as well.

3 tablespoons minced garlic
1 juiced, zested lemon
5 tablespoons Dijon mustard
3 tablespoons honey
1 1/2 cups extra virgin olive oil
1/4 teaspoon black pepper

1. Place all prepped ingredients into a mason jar. Shake well. Use for salad dressing, over meats as a marinade and for pasta salads.

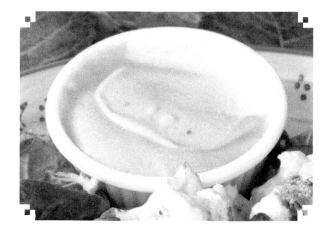

Best Home Made Ketchup

Preparation Time: 25 minutes
Cook Time: 0 minutes
Yield: 3 cups

4 dates, soaked for 20 minutes
1 cup chopped tomato
3/4 cup tomato paste
1/4 cup chopped red onion
1/4 cup agave
1/4 cup extra virgin olive oil
2 tablespoons apple cider vinegar
1 teaspoon dried oregano
1/2 teaspoon sea salt
2 teaspoons Worcestershire sauce
1/2 teaspoon black pepper

1. Soak the dates for 20 minutes fully covered by water and then drain dates.
2. Place all ingredients in a food processor or blender, blend until smooth. Store in air tight container in the fridge.

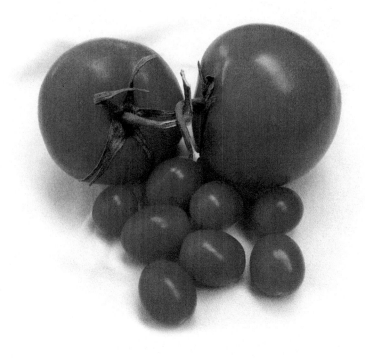

Lemon Garlic Hummus

Preparation Time: 10 minutes
Cook Time: 0 minutes
Yield: 2 pints

This recipe is super easy, delicious and creamy. Great as a dip, sandwich spread or to cook with.

1 (16-ounce) can garbanzo beans
1 (15-ounce) container sesame tahini
1/2 cup grape seed oil
2 juice and zest lemon
2 ripe avocados
2 tablespoons ground cumin
3 tablespoons minced garlic
1 bunch parsley roughly chopped

1. Drain garbanzo beans, keep the juice for the last step, place beans in food processor or blender.
2. Add tahini and pulse a few times.
3. Add grape seed oil, lemon juice, zest, cumin, garlic, avocado and parsley. Blend for one minute, then wipe down sides.
4. Slowly drizzle saved garbanzo bean juice into food processor and blend well. Serve warm or cold, delicious!

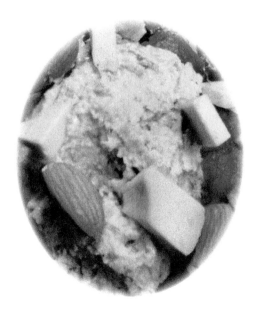

Easy Peach Jam

Preparation Time: 15 minutes
Cook Time: 30-35 minutes
Yield: 3 pints

7 large peaches
2 grated green apples
2 cups honey

1. Place a large pot with 3 quarts of water on the stove and bring to a boil. While water is heating up set up a large bowl full of ice water. Grate green apples in a separate dish.
2. Place peaches into boiling water and cook for 1 minute. Remove peaches from heat to the bowl of ice water, drain the water from the pot. To peel peaches just wipe skin with your hands and it will peel right off. To pit it, cut the peach in half and pull it apart then remove the pit. Cut peaches into small cubes.
3. Place peaches, honey and apples into the drained pot. Bring to a boil. Turn the heat down to medium and cook uncovered for 30 minutes. Stir occasionally so it doesn't burn at the bottom of the pan.
4. After 30 minutes, remove from heat. The consistency choice is up to you. Leave it chunky as is. Just the back of a fork for a little less chunky. I use a hand mixer, blender or food processor to make it smooth.
5. Ladle into mason jars. You should get 3 full jars. Refrigerate.

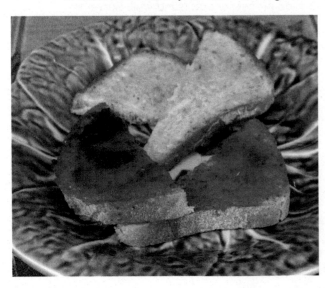

Easy Strawberry Jam

Preparation Time: 10 minutes
Cook Time: 30-35 minutes
Yield: 2 pints

2 pounds or 2 pints, halved strawberries
2 green apples, grated
1 1/2 cups honey
1 lemon juice

1. Place all ingredients into a large pot. Bring to a boil, then lower to medium heat and simmer for 30-35 minutes. Stirring occasionally.
2. Leave chunky or use a hand blender, blender or food processor to smooth out the jam.
3. Ladle into mason jars and refrigerate.

Kale Pesto

Preparation Time: 10 minutes
Cook Time: 0 minutes
Yield: 1 pint

Add more extra virgin olive oil if you desire a runnier pesto.

4 cups fresh basil
2 cups fresh kale
1/4 cup walnuts
1/2 cup pine nuts
3 tablespoons (8-9 cloves) garlic
1 teaspoon black pepper
1 1/4 cups extra virgin olive oil
1 cup Parmesan cheese

1. Add all ingredients except the extra virgin olive oil to food processor or blender and blend until smooth. Slowly drizzle in extra virgin olive oil until it's the desired thickness. Make sure to wipe down the sides as well and blend a second time.

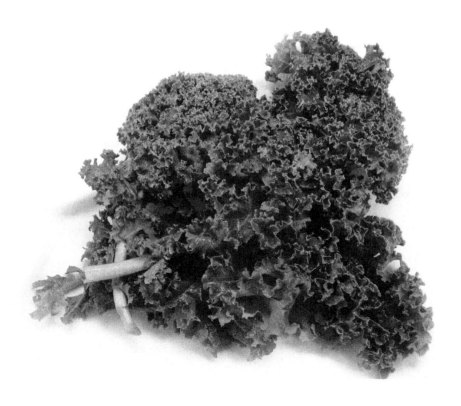

Off the Ranch Spicy Dressing

Preparation Time: 5 minutes
Cook Time: 0 minutes
Yield: 1 pint

1 cup plain Greek yogurt
1/2 cup sour cream
2 teaspoons dried chives
1 1/2 teaspoons dried parsley
1/4 teaspoon dried dill
1 tablespoon garlic powder
1 tablespoon onion powder
1/8 teaspoon salt
1/8 teaspoon black pepper
1/2 teaspoon apple cider vinegar
1/2 teaspoon agave nectar
1/2 teaspoon Dijon mustard

1. Mix all ingredients in a mixing bowl. Adjust salt and pepper to your liking. Serve with your favorite veggies and salads

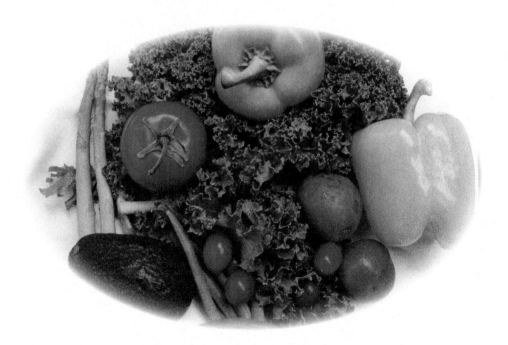

Creamy & Tangy Veggie Dip

Preparation Time: 10 minutes
Cook Time: 0 minutes
Yield: 1 pint

1/2 cup plain Greek yogurt
1 cup sour cream
1 teaspoon Worcestershire sauce
2 teaspoons dill weed
1 teaspoon black pepper
1 teaspoon garlic powder
1 tablespoon dried parsley
2 tablespoons apple cider vinegar
1/4 cup jalapeño juice (from jar)
1 teaspoon Dijon mustard
1/2 lemon juice
1 tablespoon salt

1. In a bowl, mix all ingredients until incorporated. Keep in mason jar in the fridge. Use as a dip or a dressing.

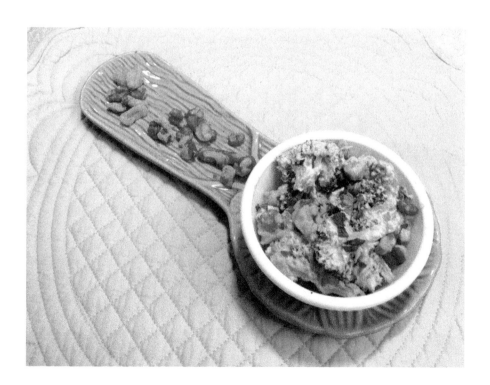

Spicy Cilantro Lime Hummus

Preparation Time: 15 minutes
Cook Time: 0 minutes
Yield: 2 pints

This hummus is creamy, refreshing and has a wonderful spiciness to it. Great for a dip, on nachos, burritos, tacos or warmed up.

1 (16-ounce) can garbanzo beans
1 (15-ounce) container sesame tahini
1/2 cup grape seed oil
2 juice lime
1 bunch cilantro roughly chopped
1 tablespoon minced garlic
2 teaspoons ground cumin
1 cup jalapeño slices (from jar)
1 cup jalapeño juice (from jar)

1. Drain the garbanzo beans, keep the juice.
2. Add the beans and tahini to a food processor or a blender. Pulse about 10 times.
3. Add grape seed oil, lime juice, cilantro, garlic, cumin and jalapeños and jalapeño juice. Blend for one minute.
4. Slowly drizzle the garbanzo bean juice in. Wipe down the sides and blend well. Serve warm or cold.

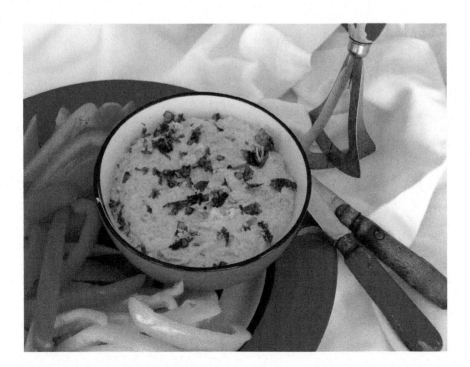

New World Marinara

Preparation Time: 5 minutes
Cook Time: 15 minutes
Yield: 1 ½ mason jars

I don't use salt much in my cooking so feel free to add salt to your taste. Also to lessen the spiciness, use less black pepper.

3 tablespoons extra virgin olive oil
3 tablespoons minced garlic
1 (28-ounce) can diced tomatoes
3 tablespoons tomato paste
2 tablespoons dried basil
2 tablespoons dried parsley
1 tablespoon dried oregano
1 tablespoon black pepper
1 to taste salt

1. Add all ingredients to a large sauce pan. Bring to a boil. Reduce to simmer, let simmer 15 minutes.
2. Leave as is or use a blender or food processor to smooth out.
3. Serve immediately warm, or store in mason jars in the fridge.

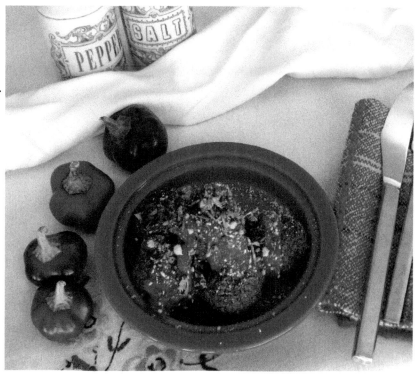

Sweet Ginger Yogurt Sauce

Preparation Time: 5 minutes
Cook Time: 0 minutes
Yield: ½ cup

This is so simple but really adds sweetness to anything you choose. It has a little gritty texture from the seasonings, but when used for a dip or sauce it shouldn't be noticeable.

4 ounces plain Greek yogurt
2 tablespoons agave nectar
1 teaspoon ground cinnamon
1/2 teaspoon ground ginger

1. Mix all ingredients together.
2. Serve as a side for dipping fruit, or drizzle over berries, oatmeal, ice cream, french toast, etc. Keep refrigerated.

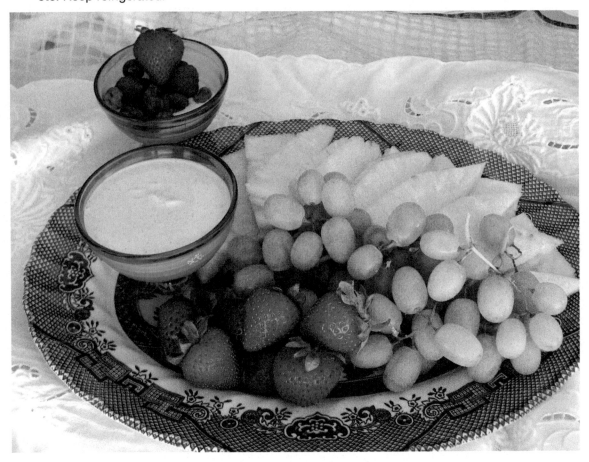

Entrées

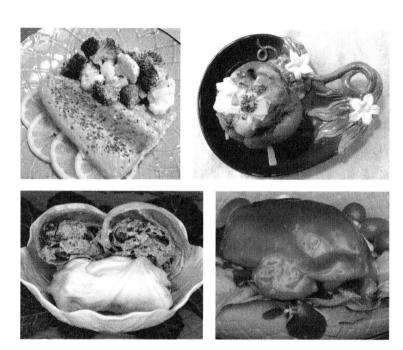

Crispy Cauliflower "Flatbread" Pizza

Preparation Time: 15 minutes
Cook Time: 28-32 minutes
Yield: 8-10 slices

Be careful with how thick the crust is for bake time, and the amount of cheese you have on top. My first couple tries the middle wasn't cooked enough.

1 prepared **Cauliflower Garlic Bread (p. 58)** Crust
1/3 cup **New World Marinara (p. 33)**
3/4 cup mozzarella

1. Cook the **Cauliflower Garlic Bread (p. 58)** Crust in a rectangle shape 1/4" thick for 22 minutes.
2. Remove from oven, spread **New World Marinara (p. 33)** on top, then add cheese. Add any other toppings of your choice, just allow for more cooking time. Bake for 10 minutes.

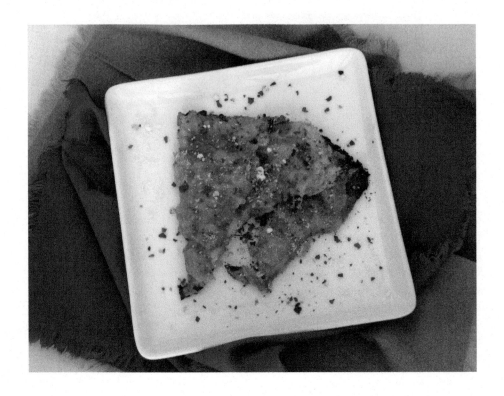

Tuna Salad Lettuce Wraps

Preparation Time: 15 minutes
Cook Time: 0 minutes
Yield: 4 wraps

12 ounces canned, drained tuna
1/2 cup **Lemon Garlic Hummus (p. 27)**
1/4 cup raisins
1 tablespoon spicy brown mustard
1 stalk celery, diced
1/4 cup diced red onion
1/4 cup grated carrot
1 large, thinly sliced tomato
1 cup grapes, halved
4 large leaves iceberg or romaine lettuce

1. Mix the tuna, hummus and mustard together.
2. Add the raisins, celery, onion and carrot and mix. Set aside.
3. Lay a large leaf of the romaine on a plate. Place 2 slices of tomato and 1/4 cup of the halved grapes on the center of the leaf. Top with a 1/2 cup of tuna salad.
4. Fold the two sides in and fold the flap facing you over to tuck under the filling and roll it up. Should look like a lettuce burrito. Serve cold.

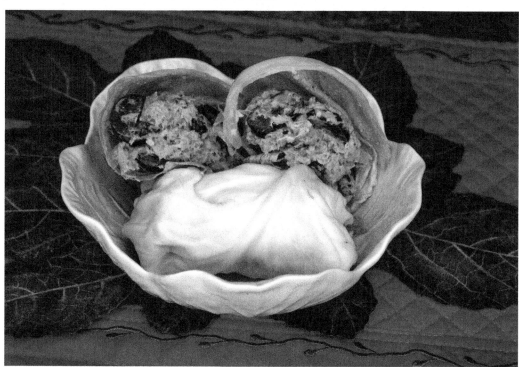

Egg-Free Eggplant Parmesan

Preparation Time: 10 minutes
Cook Time: 45 minutes
Yield: 8 servings

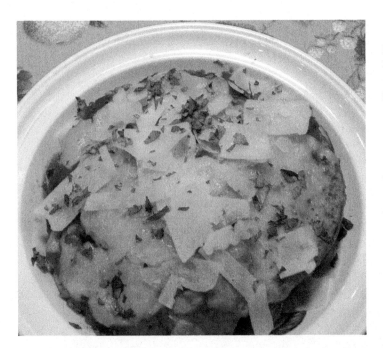

1 large eggplant, cut into 1/4"
rounds
3/4 cup brown rice flour
1/4 cup flax meal
2/3 cup water
1 teaspoon dried parsley
1 teaspoon dried minced garlic
1 teaspoon dried basil
1 cup shredded mozzarella
cheese
1 teaspoon red pepper flakes
2 cups **New World Marinara (p. 33)**
1/3 cup Parmesan cheese
1 1/2 cups gluten free crackers

1. Preheat oven to 350, grease a 13x9" pan.
2. Put gluten-free crackers in a Ziploc bag and crush with a rolling pin until very fine or use a food processor. Place cracker crumbs on a plate. Set up a plate with the brown rice flour, then a bowl with the flax meal and water mixed together, and then the plate with the gluten-free cracker crumbs. At the end of this assembly line have the greased pan ready.
3. Take an eggplant round and coat with flour, then flax meal mixture (use your finger to wipe off excess), then gluten-free cracker crumbs and place in the pan. Repeat until all rounds are done. You may have to slightly overlap the eggplant to fit them all.
4. Sprinkle breaded eggplant with parsley, basil, garlic, red pepper flakes, mozzarella, **New World Marinara (p. 33)** and parmesan in that order.
5. Place in the oven and bake for 45 minutes. Let cool for 5 minutes before serving.

Festive Shrimp Cabbage Rolls

Preparation Time: 20 minutes
Cook Time: 8-10 minutes
Yield: 8-10 servings

16 ounces medium cleaned, deveined shrimp
3 large, diced tomatoes
1 large, diced red onion
1 large lime
1 can drained, rinsed black beans
2 diced avocados
1 can drained, rinse garbanzo beans
1/2 bunch chopped cilantro
1/2 teaspoon black pepper
1 tablespoon garlic powder
6-8 large cabbage leaves
1 cup diced jalapeños

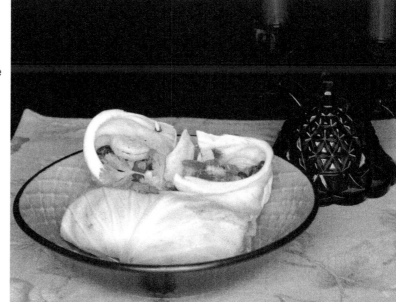

1. Bring 2 quarts of water to a boil, add cleaned and deveined shrimp for 8-10 minutes on simmer. Remove from heat, drain, and place cooked shrimp into a bowl of ice water to stop cooking and to chill.
2. While shrimps cooking begin to prep the vegetables. Take all other ingredients except the leaves of cabbage and mix in a large bowl.
3. Chop cooled shrimp, add to salad mixture and mix well.
4. Open a cabbage leaf, spoon about 1/2 cup of the salad into it. Eat like a taco, wrap like a burrito, or roll into a wrap.

Jalapeños, cheese and hot sauce are a few of my favorite toppings. Sometimes we eat it for dinner with gluten free chips. Substituting green cabbage doesn't make it less festive. It's just as good!

Hint of Pasta Veggie Salad

Preparation Time: 2 hours
Cook Time: 20 minutes
Yield: 10 servings

10 ounces gluten free pasta
1 diced yellow bell pepper
1 diced red bell pepper
1 bag frozen green peas
1 pound fresh asparagus cut into thirds
1 pound or 1 pint, halved cherry tomatoes
1 can drained, chopped black olives
1 ½ cups sliced scallions
1 ½ - 2 cups **Lemon Honey Dijon Dressing (p. 25)**

1. Cook pasta as directed on the box.
2. While pasta is cooking have another pot with 3 quarts of water, bring to a boil. Add asparagus, peas, yellow bell pepper and red bell pepper to the water. Simmer for 5 minutes. Drain.
3. Add all the ingredients, except scallions to a bowl. Mix well together, cover and place in the fridge for at least 2 hours. Before serving mix in the scallions.

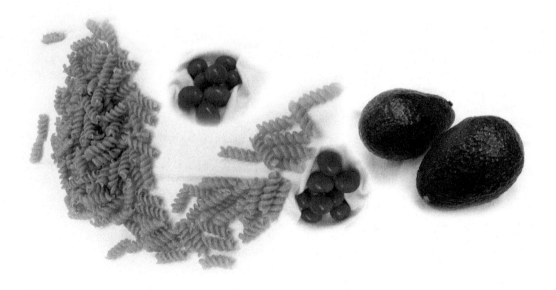

Avocado Mac'n'Cheese

Preparation Time: 10 minutes
Cook Time: 20 minutes
Yield: 12 servings

10 ounces elbow or spirals gluten free pasta
2 cloves garlic
3 avocados
1 juiced lime
1/3 cup cilantro
1 teaspoon sea salt
2 tablespoons black pepper
2 tablespoons avocado oil or extra virgin olive oil
2 tablespoons brown rice flour
1 cup unsweetened almond milk
2 cups shredded pepper jack cheese

1. Cook pasta as directed on the box.
2. While pasta cooks, Add garlic, avocados, lime juice, cilantro, salt and pepper to a food processor. Turn on for 30 seconds. Wipe down sides and mix until smooth.
3. When pasta is done, drain it and while its draining place pot back on the stove. Add the extra virgin olive oil until warmed, then whisk in the flour. It's making a roux (a thickening agent). Whisk until golden and thick. Then slowly whisk in the milk, bring to a simmer.
4. Add cheese. Stir until melted.
5. Add avocado sauce. When sauce is warmed through and incorporated, add pasta. Serve warm, doesn't hold well in the fridge.

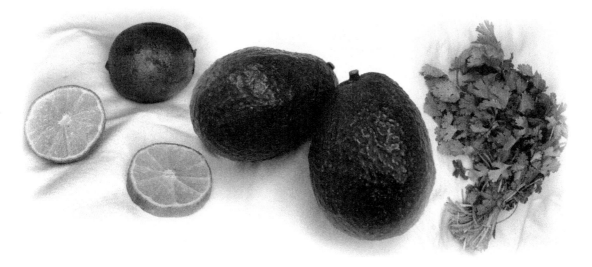

Simple Barbeque Chicken Grill

Preparation Time: 40 minutes
Cook Time: 24 minutes
Yield: 3-6 servings

3 boneless, skinless chicken breasts
3/4 cup **Over 21 Barbeque Sauce (p. 19)**

1. To heat grill: Stack a hill of charcoal in the middle of the grill. You want enough charcoal so that after it's hot you can lay it as a flat even layer of coals across the bottom of the grill. That way the heat is even on the grill. Lightly soak charcoal with lighter fluid and let sit for 10 minutes. Spray again with lighter fluid before lighting. Place lid on once coals are lit. Allow coals to turn white before spreading evenly across the bottom.
2. When the grill is ready place chicken on grill. Cover with the lid. Cook for 24 minutes and flip every 6 minutes. Brush Barbeque Sauce on both sides and cook for another minute on each side without the lid on.
3. Remove from grill to a plate and allow to sit for 5-10 minutes, allowing the juices to absorb well into the meat.

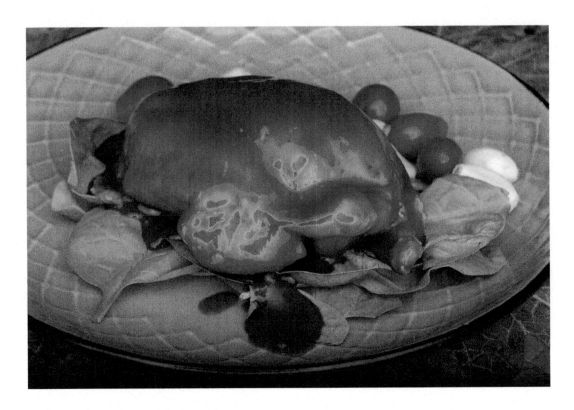

My Favorite Meatloaf

Preparation Time: 5 minutes
Cook Time: 35-40 minutes
Yield: 6 servings

1 1/2 pounds ground turkey
1 white onion, diced
1/2 cup cooked brown rice
2 eggs
1 tablespoon Worcestershire sauce
1 teaspoon dried parsley
1 teaspoon dried oregano
1 teaspoon black pepper
1-2 teaspoon salt

1. Preheat oven to 350. Grease a loaf pan.
2. Mix all ingredients together in a bowl. Form in the pan and bake for 35-40 minutes, until toothpick comes out clean.

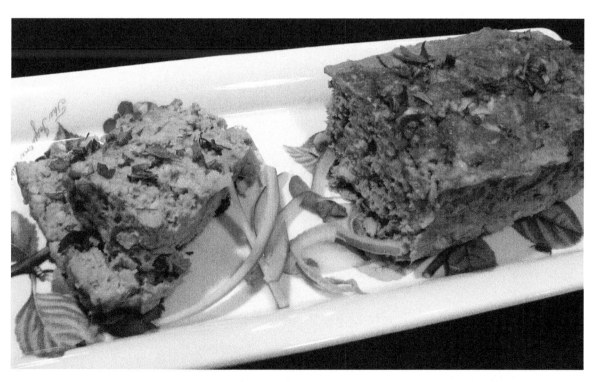

Roasted Lemon Salmon with Veggies

Preparation Time: 5 minutes
Cook Time: 13 minutes
Yield: 2 servings

Fast and easy for those on the go that want to keep it light and healthy.

2-4 ounce salmon filets
2 tablespoons extra virgin olive oil
1 lemon juice
1 teaspoon chopped basil, fresh or dried
2 cups cauliflowerets
2 cups broccoli crowns
2 pinches pepper

1. Preheat oven to 400. Grease a sheet pan.
2. Place salmon, cauliflower and broccoli spread out on sheet pan.
3. Drizzle all with extra virgin olive oil, pepper and lemon.
4. Sprinkle basil over salmon. Bake for 13 minutes.
5. Let sit for 5 minutes before serving.

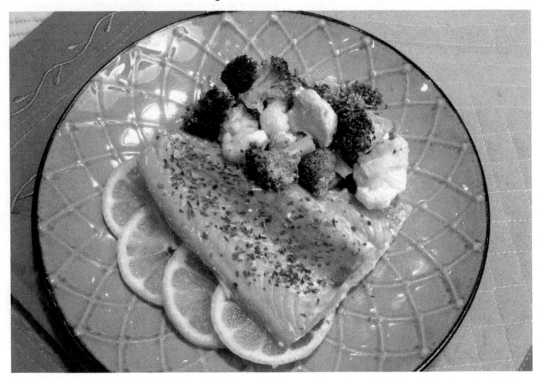

Feta Roasted Tomatoes, Zucchini and Shrimp

Preparation Time: 15 minutes
Cook Time: 40 minutes
Yield: 6 servings

6 large tomatoes, cut into eighths
3 zucchini sliced into 1/4" rounds
3 tablespoons extra virgin olive oil
1 tablespoon honey
3 tablespoons minced garlic
1 1/2 pounds shrimp; medium, peeled, deveined, cleaned
1/2 cup chopped basil
1 lemon juice
1 cup crumbled feta cheese

1. Preheat oven to 450.
2. Place zucchini and tomatoes in 9x11 roasting dish. Mix extra virgin olive oil, honey and garlic together and drizzle over the tomatoes. Roast for 20 minutes.
3. Remove from oven. Stir in shrimp, basil and lemon juice. Sprinkle with feta. Cook 10-15 minutes, stirring once.

Can be served with brown rice.

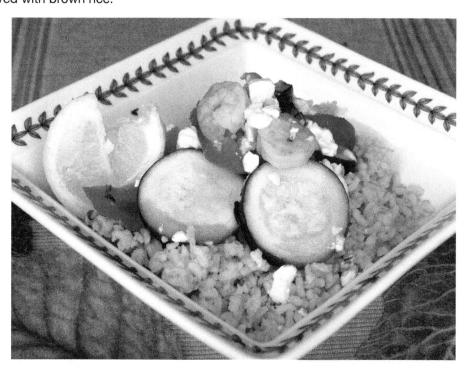

Jackie's Roasted Turkey

Preparation Time: 15 minutes
Cook Time: 3 hours
Yield: 10 servings

You can tie the back legs together and the wings down to make the turkey look more appealing for its presentation. I don't care about it so I don't do that.

1 14½ pound turkey
1 cup chicken broth
1 cup water
2 chopped carrots
2 apples, quartered and cored
2 lemons, quartered
1 tablespoon dried parsley
1 tablespoon dried rosemary
1 teaspoon dried minced garlic
1 teaspoon pepper
2 teaspoons salt
1 teaspoon dried thyme
1/4 cup extra virgin olive oil

1. Preheat oven to 325. Have a big enough roasting pan ready.
2. Remove the giblets, neck and excess skin from defrosted turkey. Stuff turkey with carrots, apples, and lemons. Place on roasting rack and put any extra of the carrots, apples and lemons in the bottom of the pan.
3. Rub extra virgin olive oil all over the skin of the turkey.
4. Sprinkle parsley, rosemary, garlic, pepper, salt, and thyme evenly over the turkey and massage into the skin.
5. Pour the chicken broth and water in the bottom of the pan. Place turkey into the oven.
6. Every 30 minutes spoon or use a baster, to pour the water and chicken broth mixture over the turkey to keep moist.
7. Cook for 3 hours or until the internal temp is 165 degrees.

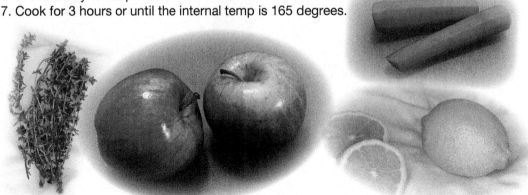

Uber Spicy Chicken Salad

Preparation Time: 15 minutes
Cook Time: 4 hours
Yield: 4 salads

3 skinless chicken breasts
1 can chicken broth
1 (8-ounce) jar jalapeños
1 head iceberg lettuce, chopped
1 (16-ounce) can drained, rinsed black beans
1 large, diced tomato
1 diced red onion
1 peeled, diced avocado
1 cup chopped jalapeños
1 cup diced cucumber
1 cup **Off the Ranch Spicy Dressing (p. 30)**

1. Place chicken breasts, broth and jalapeños with the juice into a slow cooker. Leave on low for 3-4 hours, until meat is cooked through. Take chicken out onto a large cutting board and pull apart to make bite sized pieces or shred the chicken
2. Add all prepared vegetables into a large mixing bowl. Drizzle **Off the Ranch Spicy Dressing** on top and mix until all the vegetables are covered. Separate into 4 serving bowls. Top with pulled chicken and enjoy!

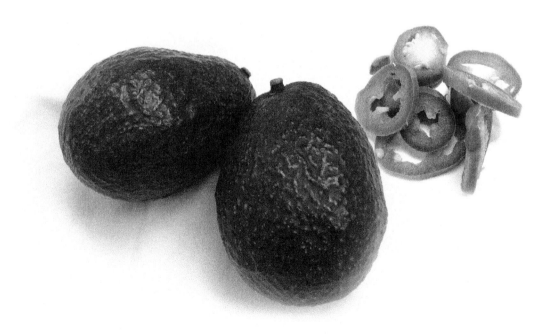

Super-Sized Spinach Salad

Preparation Time: 10 minutes
Cook Time: 0 minutes
Yield: 4 salads

I throw jalapeños in sometimes for an added spice.

4 cups spinach
1 diced red bell pepper
1/2 chopped red onion
8 ounces cherry tomatoes
1 cup broccoli crowns
1 cup cauliflowerets
1 diced avocado
1 cup raw almonds
1 cup raisins
1 cup **Lemon Honey Dijon Dressing (p. 25)**

1. Place all ingredients into a large mixing bowl, except the dressing.
2. Stir in dressing until all ingredients are covered with dressing, serve in serving bowls.

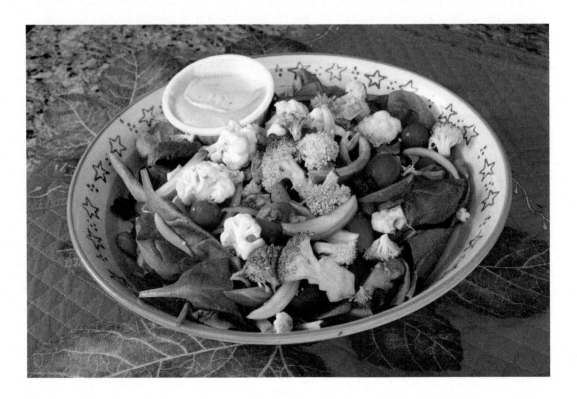

"As You Like It" Chili

Preparation Time: 10 minutes
Cook Time: 5-7 hours
Yield: 12 servings

Best chili I've ever had in my life! I turn it on in the morning and it's ready by dinner. No need to fuss. It's very versatile with toppings, as a chili cheese dip, nachos, chili cheese burgers, etc. It can also be vegetarian and vegan.

1 pound ground turkey (substitute one pound of portabella mushrooms for vegetarian)
1 large, roughly chopped red onion
2 roughly chopped green bell peppers
3 tablespoons chili powder
1 tablespoon ground paprika
1 tablespoon garlic powder
2 teaspoons ground cumin
2 teaspoons black pepper
1 teaspoon cayenne pepper
1 (16-ounce) can kidney beans
1 (28-ounce) can diced tomatoes
1 (4-ounce) can tomato paste or 6 ounce can, whatever is easiest to find.
2 (16-ounce) cans black beans

1. Chop onion and bell peppers. You want bigger pieces that take longer to cook, but not so big it's awkward to put into your mouth.
2. Add all ingredients into a slow cooker, cook on low for 5-7 hours. Amazing!

I top with shredded cheese, diced red onion, jalapeños and use gluten free chips to make nachos. Yum yum yum!

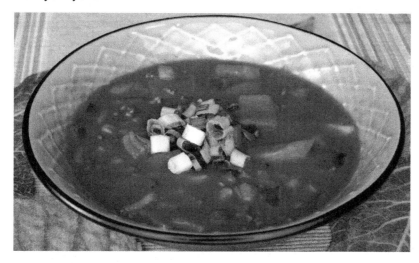

Eggplant Stuffed Bell Pepper

Preparation Time: 20 minutes
Cook Time: 22-25 minutes
Yield: 2 servings

2 green bell peppers-tops cut off, inside cleaned
2 cups cooked brown rice
3 tablespoons extra virgin olive oil
2 cups chopped 1/4" cubes eggplant
1 teaspoon minced garlic
1 teaspoon salt
1/2 teaspoon Worcestershire sauce
1/8 cup chopped red onion
2 tablespoons chopped parsley
2 dashes hot sauce
1/8 cup tomato sauce
1/2 teaspoon black pepper
2 tablespoons Parmesan cheese to add to mix
2 teaspoons Parmesan cheese to sprinkle on top

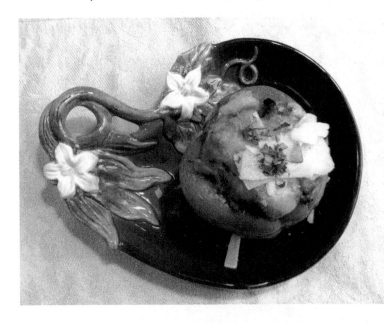

1. Preheat oven to 350. Have an 8x8" pan for baking, no need to grease. Place prepared green bell peppers on pan.
2. Cook rice as recommended on package.
3. While rice is cooking heat extra virgin olive oil in sauté pan on medium heat. Add eggplant, garlic and salt, sauté. About 8-10 minutes.
4. When rice and eggplant are cooked place in a mixing bowl, add remaining ingredients into the bowl and mix well. Stuff peppers full with mixture. Sprinkle each pepper with 1 teaspoon of parmesan cheese.
5. Bake for 22-25 minutes. Let cool for 5 minutes and serve.

Simple Veggie Skewers with Creamy Avocado Sauce

Preparation Time: 40 minutes
Cook Time: 8-10 minutes
Yield: 6 skewers

Use whatever vegetables you like as long as they will stay on the skewer after being cooked. Tomatoes get a little messy, but I still use them because they taste great grilled. This would work well with **Over 21 BBQ Sauce (p. 19)**, **Kale Pesto (p. 29)** or **Lemon Honey Dijon Dressing (p. 25)**.

4 ounces grape tomatoes
4 ounces, (4-6 mushrooms) white mushrooms
1 eggplant cut into 1/2" cubes
2 cups broccoli crowns
3/4 cup **Creamy Avocado Sauce (p. 23)**
6 each, soaked for 10 minutes skewers

1. To heat grill: Stack a hill of charcoal in the middle of the grill. You want enough charcoal so that after it's hot you can lay it as a flat even layer of coals across the bottom of the grill. That way the heat is even on the grill. Lightly soak charcoal with lighter fluid and let sit for 10 minutes. Spray again with lighter fluid before lighting, let burn until flames go out. Allow coals to turn white before spreading evenly across the bottom.
2. While coals are heating up, assemble the skewers. I did every other one an eggplant piece, but it's however and any vegetable you like. Make sure to keep some space in between each vegetable to allow better airflow during cooking.
3. Once the coals are ready place skewers on the grill perpendicular to the grill lines, so that the vegetables get grill marks. Cook 8-10 minutes with the lid on flipping half way through.
4. Remove from the grill and place on a platter. Using a brush, coat the vegetables with the **Creamy Avocado Sauce (p. 23)**.

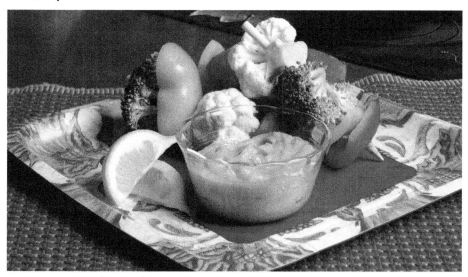

White Girl Red Curry

Preparation Time: 10 minutes
Cook Time: 15 minutes
Yield: 2 servings

Spicy and full of veggies! You can change, add or subtract any of the veggies to your liking. I would stay away from veggies that produce too much liquid, i.e. tomatoes, cucumbers, lettuces, etc.

1 can coconut milk
1/3 can water, use coconut milk can
2 tablespoons arroyo red curry paste
2 tablespoons honey
1 teaspoon fish sauce
1 red bell pepper
1 yellow squash
1/4 eggplant
1/4 broccoli
1/2 bunch Thai basil, leaves removed from stems

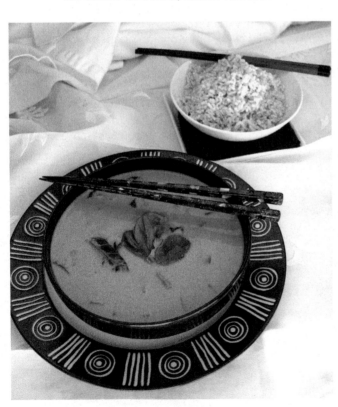

1. Bring coconut milk, water, honey, fish sauce, and curry paste to a boil. Whisking to make the paste incorporate well.
2. While that's heating up chop veggies into quarter size pieces, maybe a little bigger. You want to be able to see what each veggie is in the curry, but not have to take an awkward bite.
3. Once milk is boiling add veggies, bring back to a boil and then reduce heat to a simmer for 5-7 minutes.
4. Remove from heat and stir in whole basil leaves.
5. I like to eat this over brown rice, quinoa or couscous. Enjoy!

SIDES & BREAD

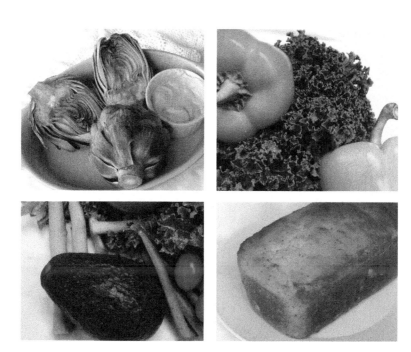

Steamed Artichokes with Lemon Honey Dijon Dressing

Preparation Time: 10 minutes
Cook Time: 25 minutes
Yield: 6 servings

2 artichokes, de-stemmed
1 clove garlic
1 sprig thyme

1. Cut about 1/2" off the thorn side of eat artichoke leaf with a pair of scissors.
2. Place artichokes in pot with water a third of the way up the artichoke. Add garlic and thyme to the water.
3. Place onto stove and bring to a boil. Reduce to a simmer, cover and cook 30-45 minutes. If the tip of a knife can punctuate the bottom of the artichoke easily, it is done.
4. Drain water, discard garlic and thyme. Serve warm with **Lemon Honey Dijon Dressing (p. 25)**.

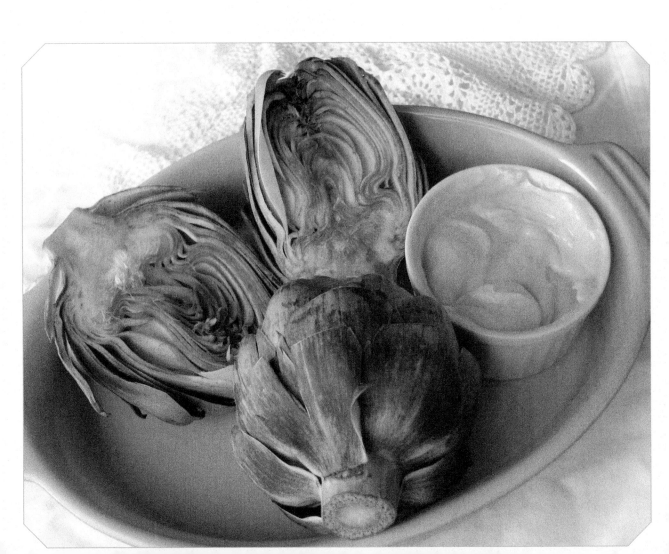

Portabella Mushroom with Avocado, Strawberry and Goat Cheese Bake

Preparation Time: 5 minutes
Cook Time: 35 minutes
Yield: 2 servings

2 Portabella Mushroom Caps
2 tablespoons extra virgin olive oil
1 sliced avocado
3 sliced strawberries
2-4 tablespoons crumbled goat cheese

1. Preheat the oven to 425. Grease a pan for the portabella mushroom caps to go on.
2. Place mushroom caps on pan and drizzle 1 tbsp. of extra virgin olive oil on each. Bake for 25 minutes.
3. Remove from oven and add 1/2 of avocado slices on each cap. Evenly top with strawberries and sprinkle with 1-2 tbsp. of goat cheese on each.
4. Place back in the oven and bake for 15 more minutes. Remove and let sit for 5 minutes before serving.

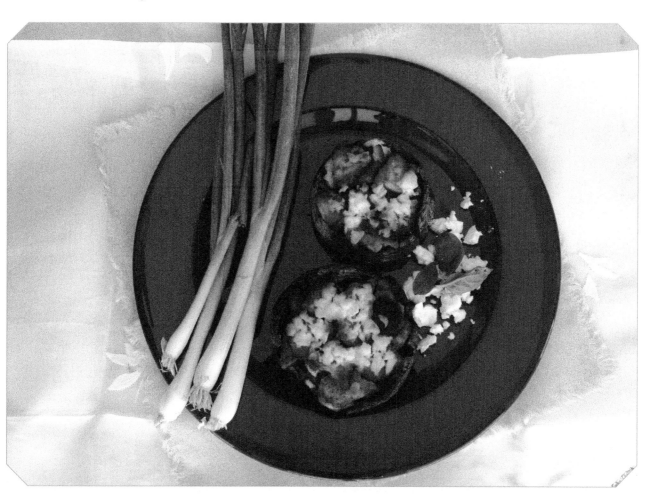

Quinoa Meat(less)balls

Preparation Time: 8 minutes
Cook Time: 18 minutes
Yield: 12 balls

1 (16-ounce) can drained, rinsed black beans
1 cup cooked quinoa
1 tablespoon dried, minced garlic
1 tablespoon dried, minced onion
3 tablespoons **Lemon Garlic Hummus (p. 27)**
1 teaspoon ground paprika
2 tablespoons Worcestershire sauce
3/4 teaspoon dried oregano
1/2 teaspoon cayenne pepper
1 teaspoon dried parsley

1. Preheat oven to 400 and grease a sheet pan.
2. In a small bowl, take prepared black beans and mash until a paste-like consistency. I used a hand mixer.
3. Add remaining prepared ingredients to bean paste and mix well.
4. Form into 12 balls, squeezing them tightly together.
5. Bake for 18 minutes. Serve with **New World Marinara Sauce (p. 33)** or **Over 21 BBQ Sauce (p. 19)**.

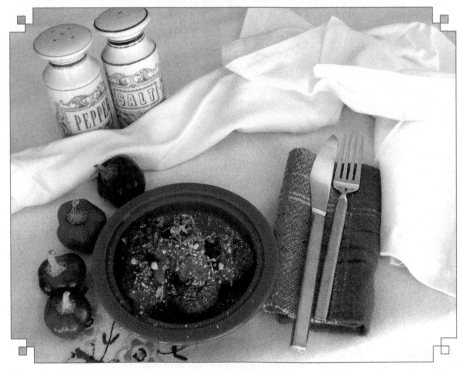

Sweet Tart Broccoli Salad

Preparation Time: 10 minutes
Cook Time: 0 minutes
Yield: 4 servings

3 cups broccoli crowns
2 cups grated carrots
1/2 cup raisins
1/2 cup chopped walnuts
2 tablespoons grated Parmesan cheese
1/4 cup **Creamy & Tangy Veggie Dip (p. 31)**

1. Mix all ingredients into a bowl. Serve chilled.

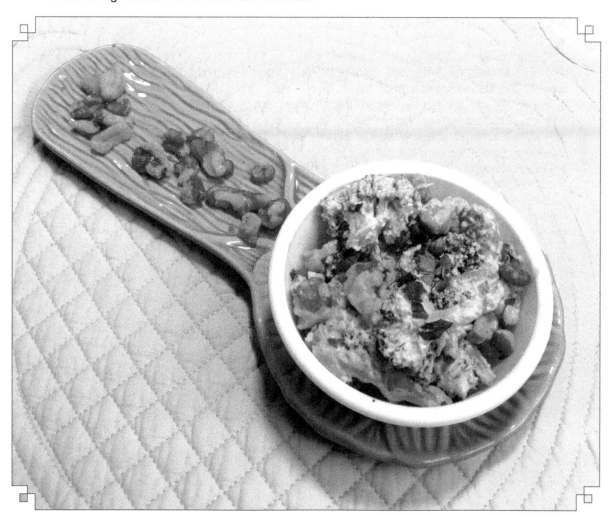

Cauliflower Garlic "Flatbread"

Preparation Time: 15 minutes
Cook Time: 22-24 minutes
Yield: 8 servings

4 cups cooked cauliflower
1 cup grated Parmesan cheese
3 tablespoons flax meal*
6 tablespoons water*
1 teaspoon dried oregano
1/2 teaspoon dried, minced garlic
1 teaspoon dried basil
1 teaspoon dried parsley
1/2 teaspoon salt
2-4 tablespoons extra virgin olive oil

1. Preheat oven to 450 and grease a sheet pan.
2. Boil cauliflower for 7 minutes, drain and place in blender, food processor or use a hand blender and blend until smooth.
3. In a small bowl and a fork mix together the flax meal and water. Pour mixture and parmesan into cauliflower and mix well.
4. Add salt, oregano, parsley, basil and garlic and mix. Spread dough onto sheet pan making a rectangle that 1/4" thick.
5. Rub extra virgin olive oil over the top of the bread and bake for 22-24 minutes until the top is golden brown. Use a pizza cutter to make slices. Serve with **New World Marinara Sauce** for dipping.
* Note: Using 3 eggs instead of the flax meal and water mixture will allow the bread to rise more.

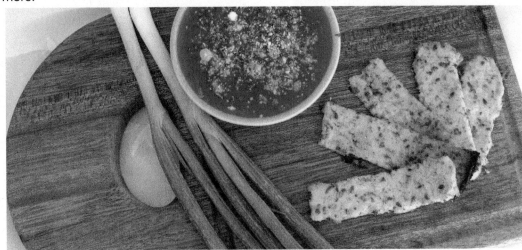

Kimber's Healthy Gluten Free Bread

Preparation Time: 1 hour, 25 minutes
Cook Time: 30-35 minutes
Yield: 8-10 servings

1 1/2 cup warm almond milk (around 120 degrees)
1/4 cup honey
2 tbsp active dry yeast
1 egg
1/3 cup egg whites
1 tbsp apple cider vinegar
1/4 cup grapeseed oil
2 1/2 cup brown rice flour
1/2 cup almond flour
1 tbsp baking powder
1 tbsp guar gum
1 tsp salt

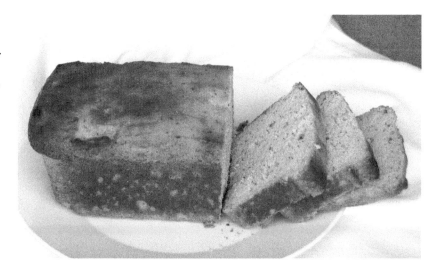

•Preheat oven to 375 and
grease 1 loaf pan.

1. Warm milk on stove
top or in a microwave.
Add honey and mix until
incorporated. Add
yeast and mix until incorporated. Let stand 10 minutes. If the mixture is foaming, the yeast is activating.
2. In a separate bowl mix brown rice flour, almond flour, baking powder, guar gum and salt.
3. Place eggs, grapeseed oil, and apple cider vinegar in a mixer bowl and mix for 1 minute using the paddle attachment.
4. Add yeast mixture to the bowl with wet ingredients and mix for 30 seconds.
5. Beat in flour mixture slowly and beat for 3 minutes once all ingredients are in the bowl. It will have a soft serve ice cream consistency.
6. Scoop batter into the prepared loaf pan and press flat, to remove air bubbles, and smooth top for a nice smooth top once baked. Leave covered with clean lint-free towel for 25-30 minutes on top of the stove while the oven preheats to help the bread rise.
7. Bake for 20 minutes. Then top the loaf with foil to stop browning too much. Bake for 10-15 more minutes or until a thermometer reads 165.
8. Let bread cool for 5 minutes in the pan and then flip out and onto a cooling rack. Let cool fully before slicing in. Keep bread wrapped to keep fresher longer.

Red Citrus Quinoa

Preparation Time: 10 minutes
Cook Time: 13 minutes
Yield: 4 servings

1 cup red quinoa
1 3/4 cups water
1 juiced, zested orange
2 tablespoons extra virgin olive oil
1/2 cup slivered almonds
1/2 cup dried cranberries
1/2 bunch sliced scallions green onions

1. Bring water to a boil. Pour quinoa into pot. Turn heat to simmer, cook for 13 minutes. Remove from heat, fluff with a fork and let sit, covered for 5 minutes.
2. Add orange juice, zest and extra virgin olive oil to quinoa and mix well. Add the cranberries and almonds, mix well. Place in a serving bowl.
3. Sprinkle scallions on top of the salad to only heat them, if we mix while it's warm it will cook them and make them shrivel.

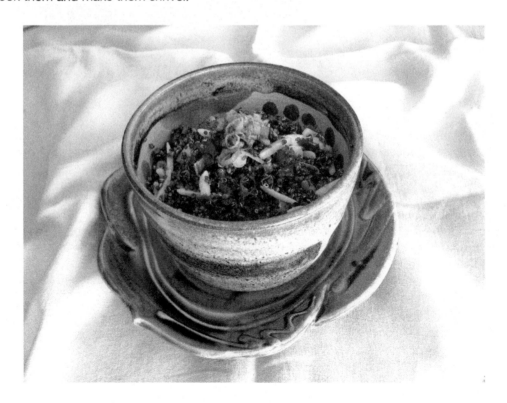

Fluffy Cauliflower and Kale

Preparation Time: 10 minutes
Cook Time: 25 minutes
Yield: 4 servings

These are low calorie and full of vitamins and nutrients. Adding 1/2 cup of your favorite cheese is a fun option.

2 cups cleaned cauliflowerets
2 tablespoons extra virgin olive oil
4 cups cleaned, chopped Kale
3 tablespoons minced garlic
1/4 cup unsweetened almond milk
1/4 cup plain Greek yogurt
1/2 lemon juice
1/3 cup flax meal
salt and pepper to taste

1. Bring 2 quarts of water to a boil (8 cups). Add cauliflower and simmer 5 minutes. Drain.
2. While cauliflower is cooking; Heat a sauté pan to med-high heat with extra virgin olive oil. Add kale and sauté for 7-10 minutes, add garlic the last minute. Remove from heat.
3. In a food processor add the cauliflower. Turn on for a minute or so, until the cauliflower is smooth like mashed potatoes.
4. Add the flax meal, lemon juice and almond milk and turn on for 15 seconds. Add Greek yogurt and turn on until incorporated.
5. Place mashed cauliflower in a bowl and stir in the garlic kale. Serve warm.

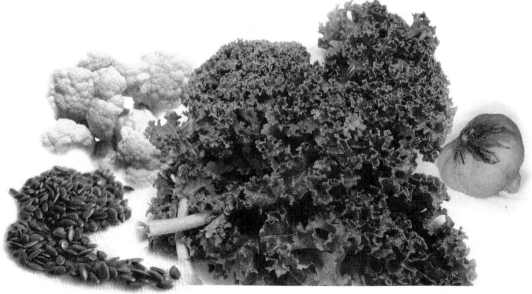

Ginger Deviled Eggs

Preparation Time: 10 minutes
Cook Time: 13 minutes
Yield: 6 servings

3 eggs
1/2 teaspoon jalapeño juice
1 tablespoon **Lemon Garlic Hummus (p. 27)**
1/2 teaspoon spicy brown mustard
1 teaspoon extra virgin olive oil
1 pinch black pepper
6 dashes ground paprika
6 dashes ground ginger
2 tablespoons chopped scallions

1. Place a pot of water on the stove with enough water to cover the whole egg. Bring to a boil, softly place eggs in pot, simmer for 13 minutes. Remove from heat and place in a bowl of ice water.
2. Peel each egg. Slice in half, lengthwise and remove the yolks into a small mixing bowl.
3. Add the jalapeño juice, hummus, mustard, extra virgin olive oil, and black pepper to the yolks and mix well. If you would like it a little less stiff slowly add extra virgin olive oil until smoothness that is desired. Evenly spoon yolk mixture back into the egg white.
4. Sprinkle ground ginger and ground paprika over eggs. Sprinkle scallions to finish. Serve cold.

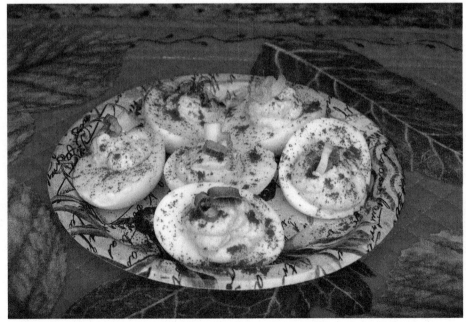

Simplified Green beans

Preparation Time: 10 minutes
Cook Time: 29 minutes
Yield: 6 servings

4 cups green beans
1/4 cup extra virgin olive oil
1/2 lemon juice
Salt and pepper to taste

1. Preheat oven to 325. Grease a baking dish. I use a 10" casserole pan.
2. Trim both ends of the green beans off. Place in a bowl. Add extra virgin olive oil, lemon juice, salt and pepper and mix well.
3. Pour into prepared casserole dish. Bake 29 minutes.

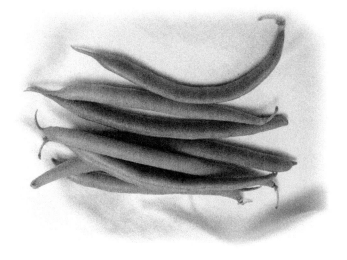

Lemon Parmesan Dressed Asparagus

Preparation Time: 5 minutes
Cook Time: 8-10 minutes
Yield: 4 servings

1 bunch asparagus
2 tablespoons extra virgin olive oil
1 tablespoon minced garlic
1/2 lemon juice
1/8 cup grated Parmesan cheese

1. Trim 1/2" off the bottom of the asparagus. Heat extra virgin olive oil in sauté pan on medium-high heat.
2. When oil is warm (if smoking it's burnt) add asparagus, garlic and lemon. Sauté for 8-10 minutes, depending on the texture you desire.
3. Remove from heat, Place on serving dish and sprinkle parmesan cheese. Serve warm.

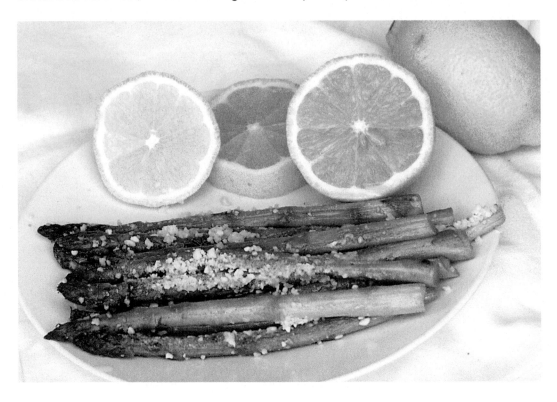

Vegan Smashed Potatoes

Preparation Time: 30 minutes
Cook Time: 5-7 minutes
Yield: 8-10 servings

5 large russet potatoes
1/2 cup grape seed oil
1/2 cup unsweetened almond milk (no vanilla added)
1 tablespoon salt
1 teaspoon pepper
1/4 cup flax meal

1. In a large pot bring 4 quarts of water to a boil. While water is heating up, cut potatoes into 1" cubes. I don't peel my potatoes but you are more than welcome to if you don't prefer the skins on.
2. Add cubed potatoes and simmer for 5-7 minutes. Poke with a fork. If fork goes into potato easily they are done. Drain.
3. Once drained, add back to the pot and mash. I use my hand mixer.
4. After potatoes are mashed, add grape seed oil, almond milk, flax meal, salt and pepper. Stir until incorporated.
5. Serve warm.

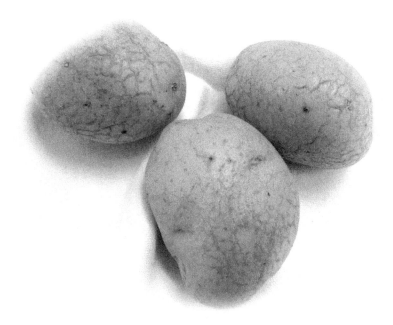

Mom and Me Potato Salad

Preparation Time: 2-4 hours
Cook Time: 13 minutes
Yield: 10-12 servings

I took my mom's potato salad recipe that I loved growing up, and made it my own with some healthy twists. You can also add 6 slices of turkey bacon or vegan bacon if you'd like. I'm not a bacon fan so I left it out. Also use more salt if needed.

5 pounds cubed 1/2", peeled is optional red skin potatoes
6 hardboiled eggs
1 chopped red onion
1 cup diced celery
1/4 teaspoon Worcestershire sauce
1/4 teaspoon ground paprika
1 cup chopped parsley
1 cup plain Greek yogurt
1/8 cup Dijon mustard
1/4 teaspoon black pepper
1-2 teaspoon salt

1. Bring 4 quarts of water to a boil. Add cubed (peeled if you'd like) red skin potatoes into pot and simmer for 5 minutes. Stab with a fork and see if it's the desired consistency you want, not too hard and not so soft it falls apart. I would say between 5-8 minutes.
2. While the potatoes are cooking have a separate pot with the eggs in it and fill it with cold water until it's just above the eggs. Place on high heat and once the water begins to boil bring to a simmer for 13 minutes.
3. Remove potatoes and eggs from heat after each is ready. Drain both and place potatoes into the refrigerator for 2-4 hours, or until cold. When eggs are cool, peel and chop, then refrigerate.
4. Once the potatoes and eggs are cold, begin to assemble. Mix the Greek yogurt, Worcestershire sauce, paprika, Dijon mustard, salt, pepper and parsley in a bowl large enough to fit everything.
5. Add the potatoes, eggs, onions, celery, and carrots to the bowl with the dressing and mix until coated. Serve cold.

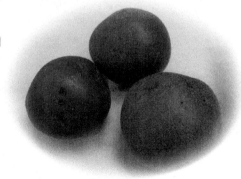

Parmesan Summer Squash Bites

Preparation Time: 8 minutes
Cook Time: 10 minutes
Yield: 4-6 servings

2 summer squash
2-3 tablespoons extra virgin olive oil
2 tablespoons minced garlic
1 tablespoon dried oregano
1 tablespoon black pepper
1/8-1/4 cup grated Parmesan cheese

1. Preheat oven to 400. Grease sheet pan.
2. Cut squash into 1/4" thick rounds. Lay on sheet pan and drizzle with extra virgin olive oil.
3. Take garlic, oregano, pepper and parmesan cheese and sprinkle each round evenly with each ingredient.
4. Cook for 10 minutes and serve as an appetizer or as a side.

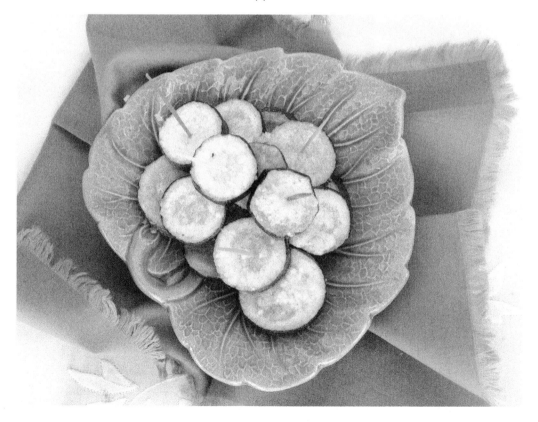

Kale Pesto Stuffed Portabella Mushroom caps

Preparation Time: 5 minutes
Cook Time: 40 minutes
Yield: 2 servings

2 Portabella mushroom, de-stemmed
1/4 cup **Kale Pesto (p. 29)**
1/4 cup shredded mozzarella cheese
1/4 cup chopped tomato
2 tablespoons extra virgin olive oil

1. Preheat oven to 425 and grease a sheet pan.
2. Place prepped portabella cap on sheet pan with the de-stemmed side up. Drizzle 1 tbsp. of extra virgin olive oil on each cap. Bake for 25 minutes.
3. Remove from oven and top with tomatoes, pesto and mozzarella evenly on each cap. Bake again for 15 minutes.
4. Remove from oven and let stand for 5 minutes before serving.

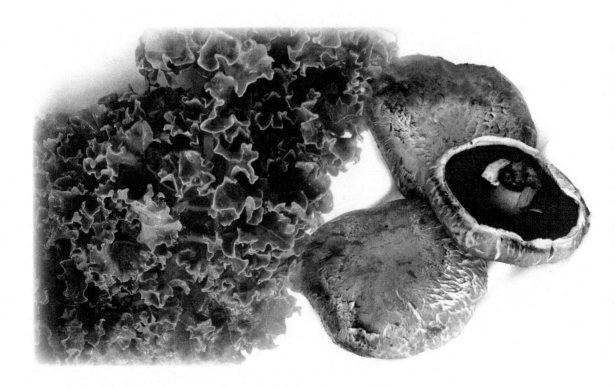

Colorful Fruit Salad

Preparation Time: 15 minutes
Cook Time: 0 minutes
Yield: 10-12 servings

Feel free to use the fruits you enjoy. It last about a week in the fridge and is a great go to for a snack. Bananas turn brown easily, but I have never minded. Raisins or nuts are a great addition as well. If you like a sauce, use the **Sweet Ginger Yogurt Sauce (p. 34)**.

1 pineapple cut into bite sized cubes
1 pint blueberries
1 pint quartered strawberries
2 cored, sliced apples
1 cup grapes
2 sliced bananas

1. Take all prepped fruit and add to a large bowl. Stir well and serve cold. Keep refrigerated.

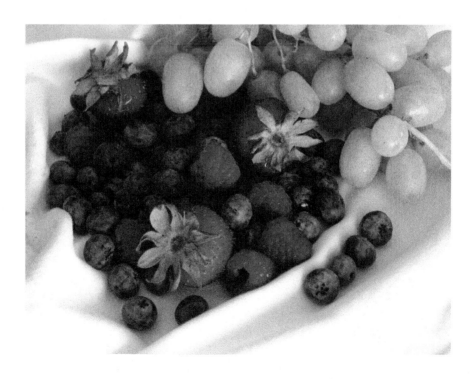

Sweet Potato and Apple Casserole

Preparation Time: 10 minutes
Cook Time: 28 minutes
Yield: 6-8 servings

Use whatever apple you enjoy, I like golden delicious but it's up to you. Also you can peel the sweet potato and apple or leave the skins on.

1 sweet potato-peeled, cut into 1/4" rounds
1 apple-peeled, cored, cut into 1/4" rounds
2 tablespoons extra virgin olive oil
1 tablespoon apple cider vinegar
1 teaspoon ground ginger
1/2 teaspoon ground cinnamon
1/3 cup raisins
1/3 cup chopped walnuts
2 tablespoon agave nectar

1. Preheat oven to 450. Grease a casserole dish, mine is an oval about 9" long.
2. Place sweet potato and apple rounds evenly in dish, alternating every other one.
3. Mix extra virgin olive oil, apple cider vinegar and agave in a bowl and drizzle over the top of sweet potato and apple slices.
4. Sprinkle ground ginger and ground cinnamon over top. Top with raisins and walnuts.
5. Bake for 28 minutes. Let cool for 5-10 minutes before serving. Smells like Christmas to me.

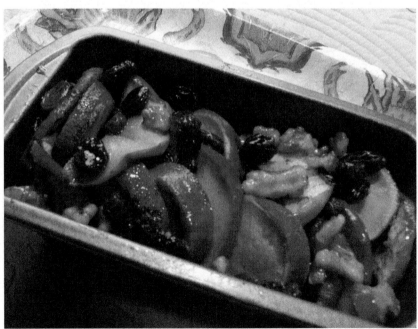

Home Baked Sweet Potato Crisps

Preparation Time: 5 minutes
Cook Time: 25-30 minutes
Yield: 2 servings

I leave my skins on, but if you're a skinless type of person go ahead and peel away.

1 sweet potato
1 1/2 tablespoons extra virgin olive oil
1 teaspoon salt
1 teaspoon pepper

1. Preheat oven to 450. Set up a sheet pan with a cooling rack on it. You will be baking fries on the cooling rack.
2. Cut fries lengthwise with sweet potatoes, 1/2" thick and 4" long, or the length of the sweet potato.
3. Place fries in bowl and toss in extra virgin olive oil, salt and pepper. Spread a single layer with the fries on the prepared cooling rack. Bake for 25-30 minutes.
4. Let cool 5 minutes, serve with **Best Home Made Ketchup (p. 26)**. Fantastic!

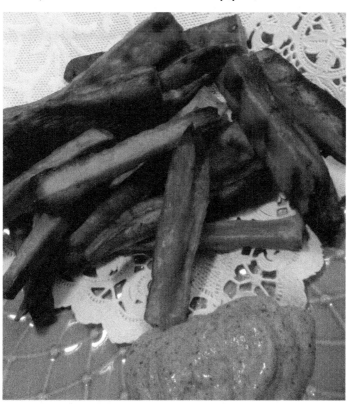

DESSERTS

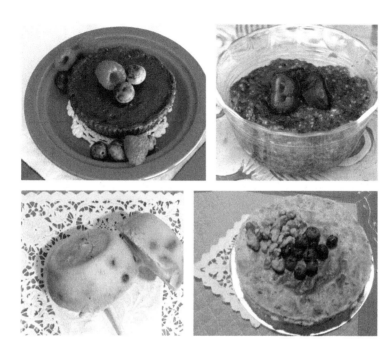

Blueberry Honey Creamsicle

Preparation Time: 5 minutes
Freezer Time: 4 hours
Yield: 2 creamsicles

I got a set of 4 popsicle containers with different color plastic lids with sticks attached from the dollar store.

1/2 ripe banana
1/4 cup unsweetened vanilla almond milk
1/4 cup plain Greek yogurt
1/8 cup fresh blueberries
1/2 teaspoon vanilla extract
1 teaspoon honey

1. Grease popsicle mold.
2. Mash the banana with a fork well. Add yogurt and milk, mix.
3. Add honey and vanilla, mix well. Fold in blueberries.
4. When spooning into the molds try to have to blueberries evenly distributed. If they are all at the bottom it might be harder to get out. Place plastic stick with a lid or a wooden stick in the middle.
5. Freeze at least 4 hours.

Strawberry Lemonade Creamsicle

Preparation Time: 4 hours
Cook Time: 0 minutes
Yield: 2 creamsicles

This has just the right sweetness and tartness. If it's a little hard when it first comes out of the freezer, don't worry it softens pretty nicely while you're eating it. If you want it a little sweeter add some more honey to it.

1/3 cup plain Greek yogurt
1/4 cup unsweetened vanilla almond milk
1/2 lemon juice
2 diced small strawberries
1 teaspoon honey

1. Grease a Popsicle mold.
2. Mix all ingredients together in a bowl with a spatula.
3. Spoon into mold, place a Popsicle stick in it. Freeze for at least 4 hours.

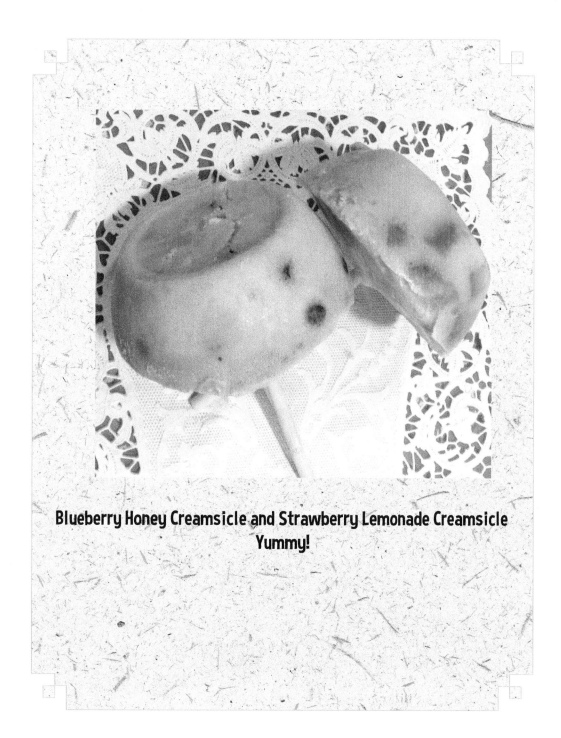

Blueberry Honey Creamsicle and Strawberry Lemonade Creamsicle Yummy!

Cinnamon Vanilla Chia Pudding

Preparation Time: 2 hours 10 minutes
Cook Time: 0 minutes
Yield: 1 quart

1 banana
12 dates
2 1/2 cups unsweetened almond milk
1/2 cup chia seeds
1 teaspoon ground cinnamon
2 teaspoons vanilla extract

1. Soak chia seeds in 2 cups milk for 2 hours in the fridge with an air tight lid. Stir well with a fork to avoid clumping. At the same time, in a separate container, mash the banana and mix it with the remaining 1/2 c almond milk. Add dates to that and let them soak for 2 hours as well.
2. After the 2 hours take chia seed mixture out and stir well. Add the vanilla and cinnamon, mix well.
3. Mash the dates with a fork, or if you need a food processor or hand mixer for a more desired smoothness.
4. Pour date mixture into chia seed mixture. Stir very well. Serve cold.

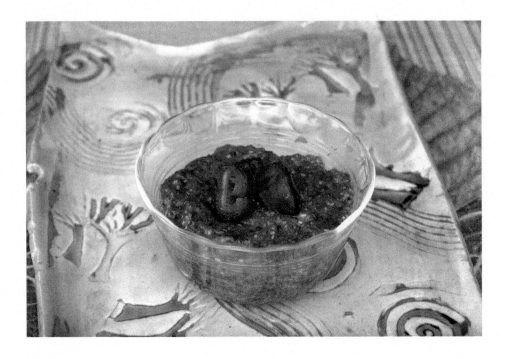

Chocolate Almond Butter Tart

Preparation Time: 2 ½ hours
Cook Time: 0 minutes
Yield: 10-12 servings

Super rich but an all-time favorite for this chocolate and nut butter lover!

¾ cup cacao powder
1 cup brown rice flour
½ cup dark agave nectar
¼ cup Coconut Oil
½ cup flax meal
½ teaspoon ground cinnamon

¾ cup creamy almond butter
¾ cup powdered stevia*

2 cups sifted cacao powder
1 cup maple syrup
¾ cup Coconut Oil
1 teaspoon vanilla extract

1. Grease and flour a large tart pan.
2. Mix the first six ingredients in a bowl together, I use my hands. Press the crust on the bottom and sides of the pan. Keep a small bowl of water nearby to dip your fingers into the water to press the crust easier. Refrigerate for 30 minutes.
3. Mix almond butter and powdered stevia together and spread over the crust. Refrigerate for 30 minutes.
4. Mix the last four ingredients together in a bowl and spread over the top of the almond butter. Refrigerate for 45 minutes. Serve cold.

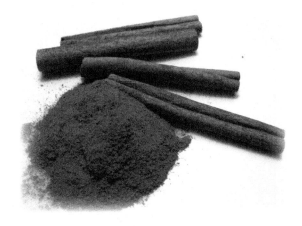

Chocolate Ginger Tart

Preparation Time: 2 hours
Cook Time: 0 minutes
Yield: 10-12 servings

¾ cup cacao powder
1 cup brown rice flour
½ cup dark agave nectar
¼ cup Coconut Oil
½ cup flax meal
½ teaspoon ground cinnamon

2 cups sifted cacao powder
1 cup maple syrup
1 cup Coconut Oil
1 teaspoon vanilla extract
1 tablespoon ground ginger

1. Grease a tart pan, and lightly coat with brown rice flour.
2. Mix the first six ingredients in a bowl together, I use my hands. Press the crust on the bottom and sides of the pan. Keep a small bowl of water nearby to dip your fingers into the water to press the crust easier. Refrigerate for 30 minutes.
3. Have a bowl of water next to you, get your fingers slightly wet and press tart crust against the bottom and sides of the pan, using as little water as possible.
4. Refrigerate for 45 minutes.
5. Mix the last five ingredients in a bowl and spread over the crust with a spatula. Refrigerate 45 minutes. Serve cold.

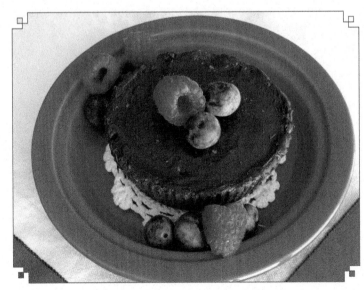

Giant Peanut Butter Cups

Preparation Time: 20 minutes
Freezer Time: 5-10 minutes
Yield: 6 cups

I use dark chocolate and almond butter, but you can use your favorite chocolate or nut butter.

12 ounces **Kimber's Chocolate (p. 87)**
1 cup peanut butter
1/2 cup **Stevia "Powdered Sugar" (p. 87)**

1. Line a 12 cup muffin tin with liners and grease.
2. Heat water in a small sauce pan and place chocolate chips in a metal bowl on top of the steam from the boiling water. Stir chocolate until it's melted and smooth. Remove from heat.
3. Doing this one at a time, with a spoon. Take melted chocolate and place about 3 tbsp. or more in 6 cups and spread the chocolate up the sides and bottom of the liners evenly. Make lids in the other 6 muffin cups by placing about 1-2 tbsp. of melted chocolate evenly on the bottom of the tin. Place tray into the freezer for 5-10 minutes to allow the chocolate to reset.
4. In a small mixing bowl, mix peanut butter and powdered stevia together. Take muffin tray out of the freezer and spoon peanut butter mixture evenly into the 6 cups. Take lids out of liners and press on top of the peanut butter, making a cup.
5. Place in either the freezer or refrigerator to store. Enjoy!

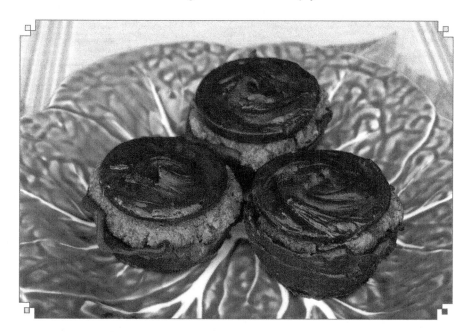

Gramma's Ginger Cookies

Preparation Time: 15 minutes
Cook Time: 10-12 minutes
Yield: 2 dozen

1/2 cup honey
3/4 cup Coconut Oil
3/4 cup molasses
1 egg
1/2 cup flax meal
3 cups brown rice flour
1/4 teaspoon salt
2 teaspoons baking soda
1/2 teaspoon guar gum
1 tablespoon ground ginger
1 teaspoon ground clove

1. Preheat oven to 350. Have a sheet pan greased.
2. Mix honey, coconut oil and molasses in a kitchen aid or with a hand mixer. 5 minutes, speed 2.
3. Add egg and mix for another minute.
4. In a separate bowl mix flax meal, brown rice flour, salt, baking soda, guar gum, ginger and clove. Add slowly to wet ingredients. About 1/3 dry ingredients at a time.
5. Spoon cookie dough on greased sheet pan, about the size of a walnut, press flat for even baking. Bake 10-12 minutes or until the bottom is a light brown.

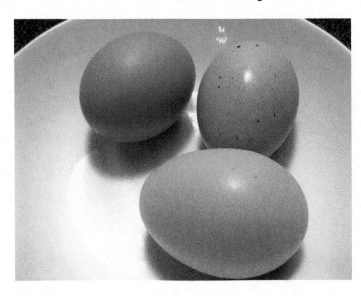

Vegan Peanut Butter Chocolate Chip Cookies

Preparation Time: 10 minutes
Cook Time: 15-18 minutes
Yield: 1 dozen

1 cup peanut butter
1/2 cup honey
1 tablespoon flaxseed
2 tablespoons water
1/2 cup **Kimber's Chocolate (p. 87)** chips
1/4 cup optional chopped nuts

1. Preheat oven to 310 and spray a cookie sheet.
2. Mix peanut butter, honey, flaxseeds, and water very well. Add chocolate chips (and optional nuts) and fold into the dough.
3. Spoon cookies onto cookie sheet, about 2 tablespoons in size.
4. Bake for 15-18 minutes, until a toothpick comes out clean. Let cool all the way before removing from sheet. They crumble easily when warm, but it makes a nice ice cream topping.

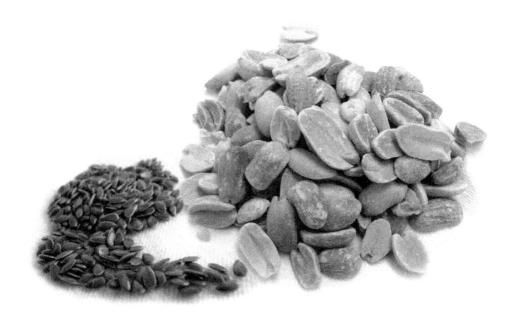

Grilled Pineapple with Sweet Ginger Yogurt Sauce

Preparation Time: 10 minutes
Cook Time: 8-10 minutes
Yield: 7-9 rings

To make pineapple rings, first cut the bottom and top off. Remove the side skin with a knife. Turn the pineapple on its side and cut 1/2" thick rounds. Use an apple corer to remove core from rounds, making rings.

1 pineapple, cut into rings
2 tablespoons honey
1/2 juice orange
4 ounces **Sweet Ginger Yogurt Sauce (p. 34)**

1. Heat inside or outside grill to med-high heat (if you want instructions on how to start a charcoal grill look under **Simple BBQ Chicken Grill p.42**).
2. Cut pineapple into rings (see note above).
3. Mix honey and orange juice in a small bowl.
4. Place pineapple on the grill and brush with mixture. Flip after 4-5 minutes. Brush the other side and cook for 4-5 more minutes.
5. Remove pineapple from grill and place on a plate. Drizzle the **Sweet Ginger Yogurt Sauce (p. 34)** over top of the pineapple or use it to dip into.

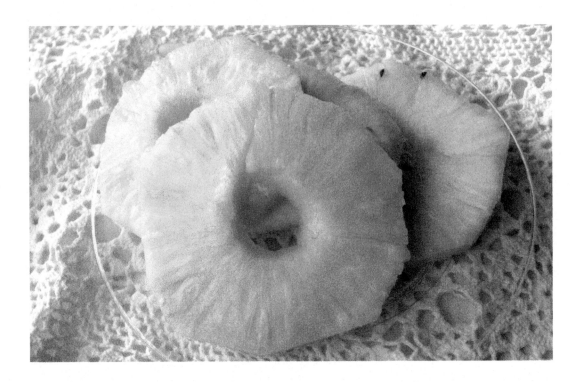

Almond Butter Oatmeal Chocolate Chip Cookies

Preparation Time: 10 minutes
Cook Time: 11-13 minutes
 Yield: 2 dozen

1 mashed banana
1/2 cup almond butter
1/2 cup agave
2 eggs
2 tablespoons baking powder
4 cups oats
3/4 cup **Kimber's Chocolate (p. 87)** chocolate chips

1. Preheat oven to 325 and grease a cookie sheet.
2. Beat (with whisk, hand mixer or kitchen aid) banana, agave and eggs.
3. Add peanut butter, mix until smooth.
4. Fold in oats and baking powder.
5. Fold in chocolate chips.
6. Spoons cookies onto sheet pan, about 2 tablespoons in size. Bake for 11-13 minutes, until the bottom is golden.

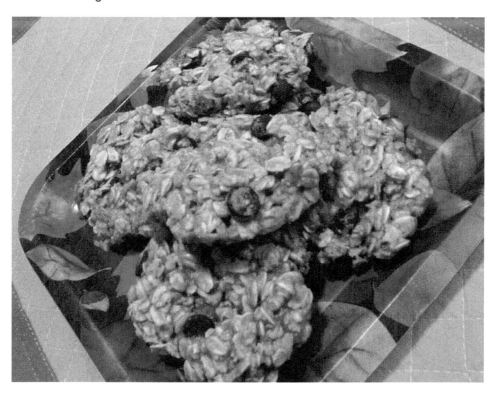

Birthday Cheesecake

Preparation Time: 20 minutes
Cook Time: 90- 105 minutes
Yield: 12 servings

1 1/2 cups walnuts
1 cup dates
2 tablespoons honey
2 tablespoons almond flour

24 ounces room temperature cream cheese
1/2 cup honey
1/3 cup unsweetened almond milk
2 tablespoons flax meal
3 tablespoons water
2 teaspoons vanilla extract
2 tablespoons brown rice flour

1. Place walnuts, dates, almond flour and honey into the food processor. Pulse, stir, pulse until smooth. Press into the bottom of a greased and flour spring pan.
2. With a kitchen aid or hand mixer, beat the cream cheese. Add the honey and beat for one minute.
3. In a bowl mix flax meal and water with a fork and add to cream cheese mixture, beat.
4. Drizzle milk into mixture, beat until incorporated. Add vanilla and brown rice flour until smooth.
5. Pour into prepared pan. Bake for 90- 105 minutes in a water bath. Refrigerate for 4 hours before serving.

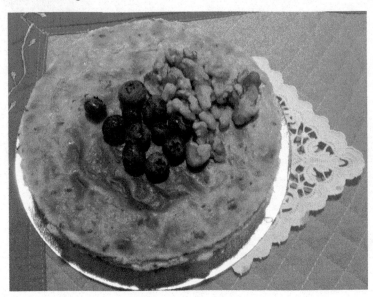

Raw Vegan Lemon Cheesecake

Preparation Time: 2 ½ hours
Cook Time: 0 minutes
Yield: 12 servings

1 1/2 cups walnuts
1/2 cup soft, about 8 dates
2 tablespoons honey
1 tablespoon almond flour

3 cups raw cashews
1/4 cup agave
1/4 cup lemon juice
1 zested lemon
2 teaspoons vanilla extract
1/2 cup melted Coconut Oil

1. Place cashews in container covered in water overnight to allow them to soften. Put walnuts, honey, almond flour and dates in a food processor and blend until smooth. Press crust onto a greased cheesecake pan. Place into freezer while making the filling.
3. Drain cashews and put into clean food processor with agave, lemon juice, lemon zest, vanilla and coconut oil. Blend until smooth.
4. Spread the filling into the crust. Wrap air tight and freeze for 2 hours. Place in the fridge. Fruit sauces go great with this cheesecake.

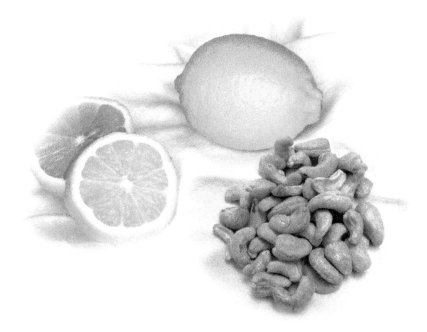

Amazingly Rich Chocolate Chia Pudding

Preparation Time: 2 hours 10 minutes
Cook Time: 0 minutes
Yield: 10-12 servings

I am in love with this dessert. I am a dark chocolate fanatic and this is filled with anti-aging antioxidants, energy boosting vitamins, speeds up metabolism, helps you stay fuller longer, and taste amazing. Every girls dream.

3 3/4 cups dark chocolate almond milk
2/3 cup chia seeds
18 (2 cups) soft whole dates
3 tablespoons powdered unsweetened cocoa
2 mashed bananas
1 tablespoon almond extract

1. Soak chia seeds in 3 cup almond milk for 2 hours. Also soak mashed bananas, 3/4 cup chocolate almond milk and dates for the 2 hours in a separate bowl. Stir a few times to prevent clumping and make sure the cover is tight to prevent a skin from forming.
2. Stir in cocoa and almond extract to the chia seed mixture.
3. Mash dates well, a fork works or a food processor. Stir into chia seed mixture well.
4. Serve with cold and enjoy!

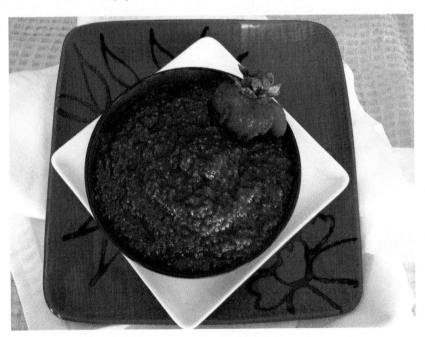

Stevia "Powdered sugar"

Preparation Time: 5 minutes
Cook Time: 0 minutes
Yield: 2 cups

No sugar for this baking staple. I love the substitute and it's so easy. It looks just like powdered sugar!

2 cups arrowroot starch
2 teaspoons powdered stevia*

1. Mix both ingredients together in a bowl with a fork. Store in an air tight container.

Kimber's Chocolate

Preparation Time: 2-2.25 hours
Cook Time: 0 minutes
Yield: 2 pints

I have made a chocolate recipe for this dessert section that is sugar free and can be chopped up into chocolate chips for use in the recipes.

1 cup coconut oil
2 cups cocoa powder
1/2 cup agave
1 teaspoon stevia powder

1. Heat coconut oil on the stove in a medium sized sauce pan, until oil becomes liquid, remove from heat.
2. Add cocoa powder, agave and stevia until well combined. Stir with a whisk.
3. Spread chocolate into a glass pan and place in the refrigerator until cooled. About 1.5-2 hours, depending on how thick the chocolate is.
4. Chop chocolate into chunks to use as chocolate chips in baking recipes or eat like a chocolate bar. If you feel like making chocolate chips you can use a small piping bag with the tip of your choice, and pipe little dots on a piece of parchment paper. Place in the fridge for 1 hour and then take them off and use immediately or keep stored in a cool airtight place.

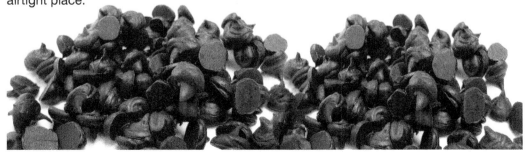

Nutty Oatmeal Raisin Protein Cookies

Preparation Time: 10 minutes
Cook Time: 11-13 minutes
Yield: 2 dozen

3/4 cup **Quick and Easy Fresh Applesauce (p. 89)**
1/2 cup almond butter
1/2 cup honey
2 eggs
2 tablespoons baking powder
4 cups oats
3/4 cup raisins
1/4 cup chopped nuts

1. Preheat oven to 325 and grease a cookie sheet.
2. In a kitchen aid or with a hand mixer, mix **Quick and Easy Fresh Applesauce (p. 89)**, honey and almond butter on medium speed for 3 minutes.
3. Add eggs, one at a time, and mix for another minute.
4. Add oats and baking powder and stir with a spoon until it's incorporated.
5. Fold in raisins and nuts. Spoon cookies onto prepped sheet pan. About 2 tablespoons worth for each cookie.
6. Bake for 11-13 minutes, or until the bottom is golden brown.

This recipe is delicious without the nuts too.

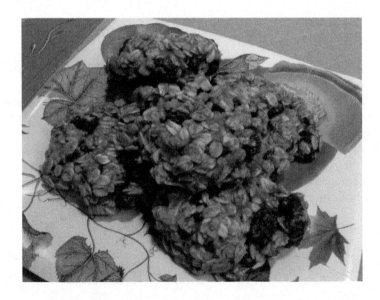

Quick and Easy Fresh Applesauce

Preparation Time: 10 minutes
Cook Time: 20 minutes
Yield: 1 ½ mason jars

You can use any apple that you enjoy eating. The green apples have the most pectin, which is a binder, so it will hold the best. I use golden delicious because of the sweetness.

4 apples-peeled, cored, and chopped
1/4 cup honey
3/4 cup water
1/2 teaspoon ground cinnamon

1. In a sauce pan, combine all prepped ingredients. Cover and simmer for 15-20 minutes. Stirring occasionally.
2. When apples are soft, remove from heat, blend in a food processor or blender. Enjoy!

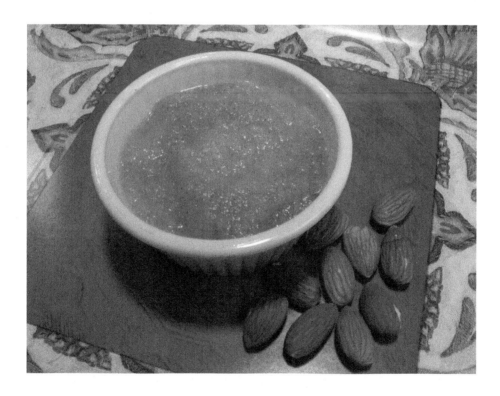

Melt-in-your-mouth No Bake Cookies

Preparation Time: 35 minutes
Cook Time: 15 minutes
Yield: 2 dozen

These are so delicious and healthy it's ridiculous!

2 cups honey
1/4 cup plain Greek yogurt
1/2 cup unsweetened almond milk
4 cups oats
1/2 cup peanut butter
1/2 cup unsweetened cocoa
1 teaspoon vanilla extract

1. Bring honey and almond milk to a boil. Ladle a small amount of the hot mixture into the yogurt until the yogurt is heated through. Add yogurt mixture to pot and heat to a boil.
2. Remove from heat and add peanut butter, cocoa and vanilla until incorporated.
3. Add oats. Spoon cookies onto a sprayed sheet pan immediately. Lick spoon while warm, yum!
4. Allow 20 minutes for the cookies to firm and set up. Sprinkle with **Stevia "Powdered Sugar" (p. 89)** if desired.

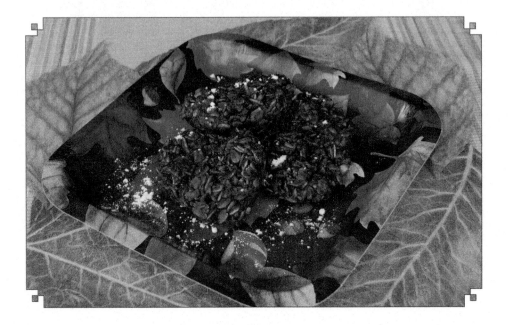

Vegan Almond Butter Brownies

Preparation Time: 20 minutes
Cook Time: 35-40 minutes
Yield: 9-16 brownies

2 (15-ounce) cans drained and rinsed black beans
1 cup dates
1/4 cup melted Coconut Oil
1/2 cup agave nectar
1 1/2 teaspoons vanilla extract
1 teaspoon salt
1/2 cup unsweetened cocoa
1/4 teaspoon ground cinnamon
1/2 cup flax meal
2 tablespoons brown rice flour
2 teaspoons instant coffee

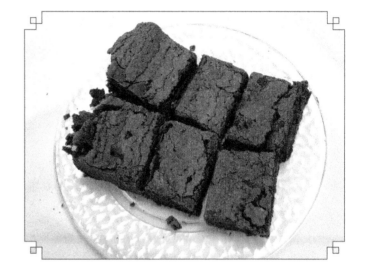

1/2 cup almond butter
1 tablespoon melted Coconut Oil
1/3 cup chopped walnuts
1/4 cup cacao nibs

2 tablespoons melted Coconut Oil
2 tablespoons brown rice flour

1. Preheat oven to 375, rub down an 8x8" pan with 2 tablespoons melted coconut oil, then lightly coat with 2 tablespoons brown rice flour.
2. Add dates, black beans, agave, salt, vanilla, and ¼ cup coconut oil to food processor or blender. Pulse a few times, and then blend for 30 seconds. Wipe down the sides and blend for a minute, or until smooth.
3. In another large bowl add cocoa, flax meal, cinnamon, coffee and 2 tablespoons brown rice flour and mix with a fork. Mix into wet ingredients, a third of the dry at a time.
4. Pour into pan. Press down with fingers. (Having a warm cup of water near you, you can dip your fingers into, and then press; helps keep it smooth.)
5. In a small bowl mix 1 tablespoon coconut oil, almond butter, cacao nibs and nuts until incorporated. Spread over the top of the brownie.
6. Bake for 35-40 minutes, until a toothpick comes out clean. Let cool. Keep refrigerated.

Nutrition Nerd

Sugars

There is so much conflicting information about the different sugars taken in through our daily foods and how they are used for good or bad in the body, that I won't go to great lengths or detail about it except to say that I learned that getting my sugars from whole foods like fruits, vegetables and gluten free grains makes better nutritional sense than any of the processed sugars and boxed foods. I use as little prepared food as possible to avoid introducing processed sugars, gluten, soy and foods that are of dietary concern. I feel strongly about my decisions due how much better I feel and the huge increase in energy I have and continue to enjoy.

Xanthan Gum vs. Guar Gum

When baking breads, muffins, scones, or other baked goods, gluten is what gives the baked goods the elasticity, thickness and sticky texture when still in a dough form. Xanthan gum and guar gum are the gluten free alternatives for baking. I only use guar gum because it is plant based. It comes from the seed of a legume-like plant, also called the Indian tree. Guar gum has eight times the thickening effect than cornstarch and is high in fiber. Xanthan gum is a corn based, fermented product that gives breads elasticity and also is used as a thickener. I don't eat corn or corn products so that is why I do not use xanthan gum. It is probably the more common gluten free alternative.

Both ingredients can be found at a local grocery store. Bob's Red Mill has both and is a brand I commonly use. Xanthan gum is usually three times more expensive than guar gum. In the Morning Glory muffins you can replace xanthan gum for the guar gum. With these ingredients I would be careful measuring too much because it can make the recipe turn heavy or gummy. Don't be fooled by their names. They are simple to find.

Soy

Soy is readily available in the U.S. now more than ever. I was always confused whether it was good for me to consume or not. Yes soy is good for our bodies, when fermented. Most soy consumption in the U.S. is unfermented, which contains large quantities of natural toxins ("anti-nutrients") and creates an environment in the body that is unable to properly digest and breakdown the protein in soy. Unfermented soy can lead to a number of risks including growth problems in children, interferes with protein digestion, may cause pancreatic disorders, may cause infertility, promotes breast cancer in adult women, may cause thyroid disease, hypothyroidism, increases the body's requirements of vitamins B12 and D, increases risk of prostate cancer, the high levels of aluminum found in soy are toxic to the nervous system and kidneys, and in infants soy formula has been linked to autoimmune thyroid disease. So if you like soy, find fermented soy products or consider making your own foods and beverages.

Salt

If there is salt in a recipe in this book, it isn't much or I say to do it to your taste. I rarely use salt in the food I consume. I knew there was a lot salt in the food I was buying at stores or restaurants so I stopped adding it to my food. I carry less water weight and don't get as inflamed. Adults should avoid eating over 6g of salt a day, or about a teaspoon. It's estimated that most people consume between 9g-12g a day. Salt is good for our bodies. It regulates volumes of fluids in the body, it aids the uptake of various nutrients into cells, it helps to regulate the body's natural pH level, and it aids in muscular contraction and its plays an important role in digestion. Too much salt can lead to hypertension or high blood pressure, osteoporosis, and stomach cancer. So the choice is yours, I just wanted to show the pros and cons of consuming salt.

Chia Seeds

Chia Seeds are one of my obsessions. I eat them every day and usually as a dessert. They help you lose weight without starving your body, balance blood sugar, help prevent diverticulitis and diverticulosis, add omega-3's to your diet (they have more omega 3's than salmon), keep energy levels high, bake as a butter alternative, have age-defying antioxidants and cut food cravings. They are inexpensive and don't have a flavor so you can flavor them however you like while getting all the health benefits.

Flaxseeds & Flax meal

Flax meal is just ground up flaxseeds. I use a coffee grinder to grind mine. Flaxseeds are used to help with many digestion symptoms, such as GI tract, constipation, diverticulitis, IBS, ulcerative colitis, gastritis, and enteritis. Flaxseed helps prevent issues with the heart and blood vessels including high cholesterol, high blood pressure and coronary artery disease. Other miscellaneous uses for flaxseed are for acne, ADHD, SLE, symptoms of menopause, breast pain, diabetes, obesity, weight loss, HIV/AIDS, depression, bladder infections, malaria, arthritis, sore throat, URTI, osteoporosis, breast cancer, lung cancer, colon cancer, and prostate cancer. When applied to the skin it aids against acne, burns, boils, eczema, psoriasis, and inflammation. It is full of dietary fiber, omega 3's and helps you feel fuller longer.

Fresh Herbs

Herbs are like little power houses of antioxidants and nutrients. They are small but are more concentrated than other vegetables. The two that I use in this cookbook are cilantro and parsley. Cilantro is full of dietary fiber, iron, magnesium and antioxidants. Cilantro is effective at fighting off different types of free radicals, assists the digestive system, fights salmonella, is detoxifying to the body, works as an anti-inflammatory, reduces bad cholesterol (LDL) and increases good cholesterol (HDL). Parsley lowers risk of cancer, enhances the body's immune system, is an anti-inflammatory, fights against diabetes, colon cancer and arthritis, is high in vitamin B12, defends against cardiovascular issues, used to fight against UTI, is a great detoxifier and is full of chlorophyll.

Cacao

Raw cacao is full of antioxidants, preservation of vitamin C, phenethylamine, omega 6 fatty acids, tryptophan and serotonin. Benefits from consuming raw cacao powder, nibs or butter are weight loss, cavity prevention, and regulation of blood sugar which is beneficial to diabetes, and benefits the entire cardiovascular system. It is full of vitamins A, B1, B2, B3, B5, B6, C, E, magnesium, copper, calcium, manganese, zinc, sulphur, iron, chromium, phosphorus, omega 6 fatty acids, saturated fats, amino acids, carbohydrates, soluble fiber, enzymes, and other beneficial phytonutrients. Cacao is the highest whole food source of magnesium.

Corn

Corn is one of the most genetically modified crops in America. This means it has under gone a DNA change and can now resist pathogens and herbicides. Any animal or crop that is genetically modified can cause health issues in humans and environmental and economic concerns. Because corn has been so structurally modified, it is harder for the body to digest. I also think of it this way; if farmers feed cows (a two ton animal) corn to make them have a larger mass, why would I eat it?

Juicing

I started juicing in March of 2013 after I had my nutrition discussion at yoga school. I thought I was pretty healthy but I always felt my energy levels were down. Coffee was always a short lived energy rush and never helped sustain me all day. I now juice with organic carrots and ginger every day. If I make a fruit salad I keep the skins and scraps and make a fruit juice (pineapple skins are delicious!). I do a scoop of each powder: spirulina, chlorella, maca, bee pollen and hemp every day.

I like to grow wheatgrass once a month, manually juice it and then add a shot into my juice. I immediately feel an energy boost and clarity of thought. Since the juice is raw and the supplements are organic, raw and in powder form our bodies can absorb and disperse the nutrients quickly, efficiently and with barely any energy necessary. Leaving more energy for the body to use elsewhere and keep us energize. (By the way, I compost the debris from the vegetables and fruits in compost pile in my front yard because my dogs would get into it in the backyard. You may want to keep it away from doors and windows in order to keep the flies away!)

The best thing I ever did was start juicing daily with supplements. You can follow me on Facebook (Happie Food LLC) and Twitter (Twitter@happiefoodllc) to find out more about how to juice and get additional recipes!

Juicing Supplements

Organic Maca Powder

Maca root is an adaptogenic root that is native to the Peruvian Andes. It is great for an energy or endurance boost, relief from stress, increase in your libido, high in fiber, can promote better endocrine system, may relieve ulcers, mild depression, menopause symptoms, it is a healthy source of calcium, iron, magnesium, selenium, and seven essential amino acids. It has a sweet taste that reminds me of graham crackers. It can be added to smoothies, baked goods or used to juice with like I do.

Organic Fresh Bee Pollen

I was recommended bee pollen because I was looking to heighten my energy levels naturally. It is full of nutrients, protein, essential vitamins, minerals, enzymes and amino acids. It has powerful benefits such as increase in libido and energy, helps ward off acne, assists with mild depression, hair growth, aids indigestion, and improves blood pressure. I use the granules in my daily juice and keep them stored in the refrigerator.

Organic Chlorella Powder

Chlorella is a single-celled freshwater algae that grows naturally in lakes and ponds. It is a true superfood and a complete protein. Chlorella powder is at least 60% crude protein, contains a full balance of essential amino acids and has 10 times the amount of healthy chlorophyll as similar greens. When taken daily, it is known for boosting calcium, iron, magnesium, potassium, and vitamins A, B12, C and E. It is a great detoxifier and cleanse for the human body. It is also known as an immune system booster, hypertension relief, infection fighting power, is a cancer preventative, reduces the side effects from radiation treatment, cures chronic bad breath, lowers cholesterol and reduces the occurrence of asthma attacks. It doesn't have a distinct smell or taste to it so it is easy for me to take. I use organic chlorella powder in my daily juice.

Organic Spirulina Powder

Spirulina is another type of blue-green algae found in most lakes and ponds. It has been used for thousands of years by the Aztec and Mayans. It is a complete protein, is packed with iron, essential amino acids, gamma linolenic acid, high in chlorophyll, vitamins : B-1, B-2, B-3, B-6, B-9, C, D, A, E, potassium, calcium, chromium, copper, magnesium, manganese, phosphorus, selenium, sodium, and zinc. It boosts the immune system, improves digestion, reduces fatigue, builds endurance, is a natural detoxifier, boosts energy levels, helps control appetite, maintain a healthy cardiovascular function, supports the liver and kidneys, reduces inflammation and benefits people that suffer from allergies. Spirulina helps against radiation therapy, it also helps the body dispose of heavy metals and it may have antiviral and anticancer effects. The taste and smell are a little rough at first. I am use to it now and look forward to juicing with spirulina powder daily.

Organic Hemp Protein Powder

Hemp protein is plant based and is the most digestible protein. It has all of the essential amino acids and fatty acids the body needs. Hemp protein is great as an energy booster, and is full of magnesium, iron and manganese. The taste has a slightly nutty flavor but is not noticeable to me and you can get different flavors at health food stores.

Organic Wheatgrass

Wheatgrass has a very sweet taste to it. Wheatgrass benefits include: increase in red blood cell count, lowers blood pressure, cleans the blood, organs and gastrointestinal tract of debris; increases energy levels, stimulates metabolism, stimulates the thyroid gland, restores alkaline to the body, treats ulcers, treats ulcerative colitis, treats constipation, treats diarrhea; it is a powerful detoxifier, it protects the liver and blood, contains beneficial enzymes. When applied to the skin it can help to stop any skin irritation and itchiness quickly, soothe sunburns, scalp conditions, heal cuts, burns, scrapes, rashes, poison ivy, athlete's foot, insect bites, boils, sores, open ulcers, tumors and more. It can prevent bad breath and help tighten gums. It neutralizes toxic substances like polyvinyl chloride, mercury, strontium, nicotine, and cadmium in the body. Cancer cells cannot exist in the presence of oxygen and wheatgrass offers the benefit of a liquid oxygen transfusion since the juice contains liquid. It turns gray hairs back to the neutral color again. For radiation patients it helps lessen the effects of the radiation. It promotes youthfulness and restores fertility. I love the effects of wheatgrass. I grow my own every month and add the shot into my daily juice. I order my kits from wheatgrasskits.com. It comes with 5 trays worth and is organic. I also think it is reasonably priced and easy to grow.

Butter:

I don't use butter for several reasons, mostly I don't enjoy the taste. I also don't eat many beef or cow byproducts. I eat cheese occasionally but I try to stick to goat cheese or vegan cheese. Butter is high in bad cholesterol (HDL) and bad fats. It does actually help the body absorb nutrients more easily, so if you enjoy butter, I say eat it. I never eat margarine, it is completely artificial. It is only one ingredient away from plastic. Just add hydrogen and you, my friends, are eating plastic. I suggest butter over margarine anyday.

Gluten:

Gluten is the compound of two proteins (gliadin and glutenin) found in wheat, rye, spelt, barley, and triticate. Wheat in the U.S. today has been genetically modified and biochemically altered to mass produce. That means, wheat used by our elders 60 years ago was much healthier than today's wheat. Our bodies have a hard time recognizing this mutated super wheat and breaking it down efficiently for nutritional value in our bodies. White flour is bleached and has the wheat germ completely removed taking all nutritional value out of it. It's estimated that over 3 million Americans have celiac disease, while many more have a gluten intolerance. Once I eliminated wheat from my diet I wasn't fatigued, bloated, my thoughts became clearer, my skin cleared up, I don't get rashes, I lost weight with no change to my daily routine, my arthritis went away, my nausea went away, my raspy breathing has gone away, and I had more energy. *Wheat Belly* by William Davis has great information.

Water:

Our bodies are mostly made up of water. According to the Mayo Clinic, (for persons without medically diagnosed disorders that require limiting fluid intake,) the average intake for men should be 13 cups per day, or 104 ounces, and for women it should be 9 cups per day or 72 ounces, roughly half our weight in ounces a day. Not only is that a task within itself, but then we have to worry about is our water clean? Well in the U.S., no, most water isn't clean, and it actually contains toxins that are harmful to our bodies. We have been told for decades that fluoride is good for us in moderation, which is true. Now it is in our food, water, toothpastes, and other household items. Fluoride has been tested and proven to harm the body. In recent tests it has been proven that excess ingested fluoride destroys teeth, causes dental fluorosis, causes disorders in the brain, nervous system, kidneys, bones, reduces IQ levels, impairs proper thyroid function, and debilitates the endocrine system.

I have "water-proofed" my house. I have a water filter in my shower. When we are in steam our body pores open, allowing the polluted water into our body more easily. I have a **Kitchen Defender** water filter in my kitchen from Sweetwater LLC, where they test the water where you live and make a specific filter for your home. I don't recommend an osmosis system because it wastes a few gallons for every gallon of drinking water it produces. People actually taste the difference in the water at my house. Big Berky is also a great company for water filtration.

Raw Food:

I eat mostly raw foods daily. It's easier for my body to digest and I never feel fatigued after I do. When we cook our food we kill 100% of the enzymes and turn them into free radicals. When we eat these free radicals the body has to use energy to fight them. It causes our bodies to produce additional white blood cells, taxing the immune system, much like the body's reaction to cancer. Moderation between cooked food and raw food is key. I have more sustainable energy now. While losing weight I found this helpful, and thought I would share. I have raw options available which is how I eat a lot of these recipes.

Organic:

I always try to use organic ingredients whenever possible. Organic food increases your consumption of vitamins, minerals, antioxidants, and essential fatty acids. Non-organic food contains harmful hormones and poisonous pesticides.

Pesticides in our food has been linked to many problems such as neurological damage, cancer, infertility, nausea, vomiting, diarrhea, allergies, asthma, wheezing, rashes, ADHD, birth defects, other skin irritations and more. Pesticides can remain in the body for years and even cross through the placenta during pregnancy, placing the fragile unborn child in danger of birth weight problems, birth defects, neurological and behavioral problems, disrupted hormone function, autism and cancer. Pesticides have also been linked to infertility in males and females.

Organic produce has outstanding flavor, and is becoming much more affordable with it's popularity increase. Do your best to use organic produce when you eat and like me, and I bet you'll feel better.

Conversions & Abbreviations

tsp. = teaspoon

tbsp. = tablespoon

oz. = ounce

c. = cup

pt. = pint

qt. = quart

lbs. or # =pounds

gal. = gallons

3 tsp = 1 tbsp.

2 tbsp. = 1 oz. = 1/8 cup

8 oz. = 1 c. = ½ lb.

2 c = 1 pt. = 16 oz. = 1 lb.

4 c = 2 pt. = 1 qt. = 32 oz. = 2 lbs.

4 qt = 1 gal or 128 oz.

Substitutions

Eggs:

> 1 tbsp. flax meal + 2-3 tbsp. water = 1 egg

Baking Soda and Baking Powder:

> 1 tsp. baking soda = 3 tsp. baking powder

Sugar:

> 1 c. sugar = 2/3 c. - ¾ c. honey.
> 1 c. sugar = ¾ c. maple syrup
> 1 c. sugar = 2 bananas mashed
> 1 c. sugar = 8 to 10 dates, softened and mashed
> 1 c. sugar = ¾ c. agave nectar
> 1 c. sugar = 1 1/3 c. molasses

Butter:

> 1 c. butter = ½ c. oil (extra virgin olive oil, grape seed, avocado, coconut, peanut and so on)
> 1 c. butter = 1 c. applesauce
> 1 c. butter = 1 c. sour cream
> 1 c. butter = 1 c. plain Greek yogurt or dairy free yogurt
> 1 c. butter = 1 c. avocado mashed

Bread Crumbs:

> *Savory:* gluten free bread crumbs, gluten free crackers or bean chips chopped up in blender, roasted eggplant or raw cauliflower chopped in a blender, hummus or a hard grated cheese.

Sweet: banana chips chopped up in a food processor, oats, or your favorite granola.

Nut Butters:

You can substitute any nut butter with another. I used peanut butter most times in this recipe book because it is the most common in households. I like almond butter, cashew butter, walnut butter, pretty much all of them. I always get them raw and unsalted. Read the ingredients carefully, some nut butters have hidden Trans fats.

Flours:

There are many alternatives to wheat flour when cooking and baking. Brown rice flour and white rice flour are lighter and is best for baking. Almond flour is a little heavier and is great for crusts and coatings. The other flours you can find in grocery stores are fava beans, sorghum, white beans, amaranth, potato, oats (make sure they're certified gluten free), tapioca and millet.

All-Purpose Flour Mixes:

1 ½ cup brown rice flour
1 ½ c potato starch or arrowroot powder
1 c tapioca flour

Milk:

I use unsweetened almond milks, flaxseed milk, and coconut milk. I stay away from soy because if unfermented it can become toxic to the body, and most soy products in America are unfermented. I also avoid cow's milk, because of all the added hormones, preservatives and other toxic additives.

Honey vs. Agave

I just wanted to throw this quick note in here. Honey and agave nectar are interchangeable. They have the same sweetness, but different flavors. There are different flavors of agave nectar depending on the taste you desire. The main difference is honey is an animal byproduct and agave is a vegan alternative to sugar. Maple syrup is a little sweeter than both, and is another vegan alternative.

Recipe List by Section

(Alphabetical index with page numbers following)

Breakfast

Dips and Sauces

New World Marinara
Sweet Ginger Yogurt Sauce

Entrées
Crispy Cauliflower "Flatbread" Pizza
Tuna Salad Lettuce Wraps
Egg-Free Eggplant Parmesan
Festive Shrimp Cabbage Rolls
Hint of Pasta Veggie Salad
Avocado Mac'n'Cheese
Simple Barbeque Chicken Grill
My Favorite Meatloaf
Roasted Lemon Salmon with Veggies
Feta Roasted Tomatoes, Zucchini and Shrimp
Jackie's Roasted Turkey
Uber Spicy Chicken Salad
Super-Sized Spinach Salad
"As You Like It" Chili
Eggplant Stuffed Bell Pepper
Simple Veggie Skewers with Creamy Avocado Sauce
White Girl Red Curry

Sides & Bread
Steamed Artichokes with Lemon Honey Dijon Dressing
Portabella Mushroom with Avocado, Strawberry and Goat Cheese Bake
Quinoa Meat(less)balls
Sweet Tart Broccoli Salad
Cauliflower Garlic "Flatbread"
Kimber's Healthy Gluten Free Bread
Red Citrus Quinoa
Fluffy Cauliflower and Kale
Ginger Deviled Eggs
Simplified Green beans
Lemon Parmesan Dressed Asparagus
Vegan Smashed Potatoes
Mom and Me Potato Salad

Parmesan Summer Squash Bites
Kale Pesto Stuffed Portabella Mushroom caps
Colorful Fruit Salad
Sweet Potato and Apple Casserole
Home Baked Sweet Potato Crisps

Desserts
Blueberry Honey Creamsicle
Strawberry Lemonade Creamsicle
Cinnamon Vanilla Chia Pudding
Chocolate Almond Butter Tart
Chocolate Ginger Tart
Giant Peanut Butter Cups
Gramma's Ginger Cookies
Vegan Peanut Butter Chocolate Chip Cookies
Grilled Pineapple with Sweet GingerYogurt Sauce
Almond Butter Oatmeal Chocolate Chip Cookies
Birthday Cheesecake
Raw Vegan Lemon Cheesecake
Amazingly Rich Chocolate Chia Pudding
Kimber's Chocolate
Stevia "Powdered sugar"
Nutty Oatmeal Raisin Protein Cookies
Quick and Easy Fresh Applesauce
Melt-in-your-mouth No Bake Cookies
Vegan Almond Butter Brownies

Recipe Index

Sources

Martin-Kilgour, Zak. "Did you know the raw cacao benefits human longevity and health without negative side effects?", 2009 <www.secrets-of-longevity-in-humans.com/raw-cacao-benefits.html>

Rodgers, Joshua. "10 powerful health benefits of parsley." Natural Alternative Remedy. July 12, 2013. <www.naturalalternativeremedy.com/10-powerful-health-benefits-of-parsley/>

Cashin-Garbutt, April. "Salt intake: why is it bad for you?" May 21, 2012. www.news-medical.net/news/20120521/Salt-intake-why-is-it-bad-for-you.aspx

Martinio, Joe. "Confused about soy? Soy dangers summarized." Collective Evolution. February 21, 2013. <http://www.collective-evolution.com/2013/02/21/confused-about-soy-soy-dangers-summarized/>

Skae, Teya. "The harmful effects of sugar and choosing healthy alternatives." Natural News. February 21, 2008. www.naturalnews.com/022692_sugar_xylitol_stevia.html

Gruss, Teri. "How to use Xanthan Gum and Guar Gum in Gluten-Free Cooking". About.com, INCup 2013. http://glutenfreecooking.about.com/od/glutenfreecookingbasics/a/xanthanguargums.htm

Huff, Ethan A. "ADA study confirms dangers of fluoridated water, especially for babies." Natural News. October 21, 2010. www.naturalnews.com/z030123_fluoride_babies.html

Ward, Elizabeth M. "What to know about gluten-free flours, including nutritional information." WebMD. Kathleen M Zelman. 2012. www.webmd.com/digestive-disorders/celiac-disease/features/gluten-free-flours?print=true#

Kiefer, David MD. "Flaxseed Overview Information." WebMD. December 14, 2012. http://www.webmd.com/vitamins-and-supplements/lifestyle-guide-11/supplement-guide-flaxseed-oil

"Health Benefits of Cilantro One of Nature's Best Antioxidant Foods." 2009-2013. http://www.antioxidants-for-health-and-longevity.com/benefits-of-cilantro.html

"Benefits of Wheatgrass." 2013. Hippocrates Health Institute. http://www.hippocratesinst.org/wheatgrass/benefits-of-wheatgrass

Jeffery. "Maca Powder", "Bee Pollen Granules", "Chlorella Powder", "Spirulina Powder", "Whole Hemp Seeds", and " Chia Seeds" Nuts.com. 1999-2013. www.nuts.com/cookingbaking/powders/organic-maca-powder/premium.html, <www.nuts.com/cookingbaking/powders/beepollen/granules.html>, www.nuts.com/cookingbaking/powders/chlorella/organicuphtml, www.nuts.com/cookingbaking/powders/spirulina/organicuphtml, www.nuts.com/cookingbaking/seeds/hemp/wholesale.html, www.nuts.com/cookingbaking/chia-seeds/premium.html.

Chalt, Jennifer. "8 reasons why consumers should buy organic food." About.com. 2013. http://organicupabout.com/od/OrganicConsumerRelations/tp/8-Reasons-Why-Consumers-Should-Buy-Organic-Food.htm

Mayo Clinic— Mayo Foundation for Medical Education and Research. "Water: How much should you drink every day?" http://www.mayoclinic.org/healthy-living/nutrition-and-healthy-eating/in-depth/water/art-20044256 depth/water/art-20044256

Recommended Books & Documentaries

Books:

Davis, William, *Wheat Belly* (Rodale Press, 2011).
Brazier, Brendan, *Thrive* (Da Capo Press, Perseus Books Group, 2007).
Campbell PhD, T. Colin and Campbell II MD, Thomas M. *The China Study* (BenBella Books, 2005).

Documentaries:

Happy, Dir: Roko Belic, 2011.
Food Matters, Dir: James Colquhoun, Carlo Ledesma, 2008.
Vegucated, Dir: Marisa Miller Wolfson, 2011.
Food, Inc., Dir: Robert Kenner, 2008.

Afterthoughts

I first knew I wanted to be healthy at age seventeen. I was brought up in a family that consumed a lot of fast foods, frozen meals, and processed foods that lasted forever in the pantry. When I decided I wanted to live a healthier lifestyle I had no one to direct or educate me. The first things to go were soda and fast food. Gradually I learned what to eliminate from my diet and what worked for my body.

I loved baking and cooking with my grandma as a child and teenager. Gramma always made our time in the kitchen fun and the people we cooked for were always happier after the meal. Our food wasn't the healthiest, but the positive feeling food brought to everyone was the deciding factor when choosing my career. I began to research nutrition on my own. And that is how my journey to Happy Food began. In 2008 graduated from California Culinary Academy where I learned my skill as a chef.

I stopped eating processed sugar in 2012 to see how I felt and the results were amazing. I stopped having crashes during the day. I felt energized all day long, my cravings for sugar and carbs went away and I wasn't as moody. In 2013, after reading *Wheat Belly* by Dr. William Davis, I challenged myself to remove gluten from my diet for a year. Afterwards, I became allergic to gluten. Now I get incredibly sick when I eat or come into contact with gluten. I don't agree with the way animals are processed from pasture to table so I've stopped consuming all meat products that are raised with these cruel practices. I am alarmed by the toxins and hormones used in preparing bulk meat for stores these days. I eat seafood and chicken when I know where and how it has been raised and processed, which can be tough at times. Since changing my diet I have lost forty pounds and dropped ten pant sizes.

I know first-hand how lonely it feels to be overweight and unhealthy. But we don't have to be alone in this fight. We can unite and make this country supply our demand for healthy food through our choices at our markets. Never forget your power as a consumer and your power with your thoughts.

Believe in yourself and others, and you can do and be whatever you want to be.

I am just here as a guide to help you on your journey.

CPSIA information can be obtained at www.ICGtesting.com
Printed in the USA
LVOW02s1318210615

443276LV00006B/7/P